The Emergency Practitioner's Handbook

for all front line health professionals

Mary Dawood
Nurse Consultant in Emergency Medicine,
Imperial College Healthcare Trust,
London, UK

Foreword by

Robin Touquet
Emeritus Professor of Emergency Medicine,
Imperial College, London, UK and Locum Consultant,
Kingston NHS Trust

Radcliffe Publishing
London • New York

Radcliffe Publishing Ltd
33–41 Dallington Street
London
EC1V 0BB
UK
www.radcliffepublishing.com

British Library Cataloguing in Publication Data

A catalogue record for this book is available from the British Library.

ISBN-13: 978 184619 404 7

The paper used for the text pages of this book is FSC certified. FSC (The Forest Stewardship Council) is an international network to promote responsible management of the world's forests.

Typeset by Phoenix Photosetting, Chatham, Kent, UK
Cover designed by Cox Design Ltd, Witney, Oxon, UK
Printed and bound by TJ International Ltd, Padstow, Cornwall, UK

Contents

Foreword

This is *the* book for all those who work in, or are responsible for, the 'minors' area of emergency departments, or nurse-led minor injuries unit (or whatever title is given). 'Minors' is actually a dangerous name, for in 'minors' not only are most patients discharged home, usually without seeing an emergency medicine consultant, but serious pathology may be seen in its early stages, all too easily wrongly triaged! 'Minors' necessitates prompt detection, delineation and, where appropriate, referral. It is not 'easy street'.

Nurse core training is not based initially on making definitive diagnoses by history, examination or special investigation. Junior doctors, whilst comfortable working with major patients, may be all at sea in 'minors'. The general practitioner may not directly have reviewed X-rays, nor have assessed 'minor' trauma, since VTS training.

A patient discharged home with a missed division of a tendon or a nerve may sue for large sums by way of compensation. Missed early infection (e.g. malaria), sepsis or delirium may result in death. Extra vigilance is required for children and the elderly.

The emergency practitioner (of whatever discipline) must practise to a standard to be expected of their rank, training and qualifications but with the caveat that, when in doubt, help must be asked for. This standard is 'the reasonable standard' – not necessarily the best standard (for no one is perfect, although we all must be safe) – to be expected of a nurse practitioner, junior hospital doctor (often a Foundation Year 2 doctor, FY2) or general practitioner. The greater the inexperience, the lower must be the threshold for asking for advice. It is not always easy to make that decision; once made, the presenting pathology must be focused into an articulate referral or call for help.

Mary Dawood and her collaborators have laid down with logic, reason and balance what is this reasonable standard. Thereby patients will be given a consistent standard of care, whoever is caring for them.

Therefore this book is timely and a 'must read' for all those who are starting out in 'minors', be they a nurse, junior doctor or general practitioner. The senior nurse may be much more comfortable working in 'minors' than the junior doctor, who must therefore be especially careful, even humble.

No minor injuries unit or area (within an emergency department) can work in isolation. Emergency medicine specialists (consultants and associate specialists), and their trainees, must understand what standards to expect from their 'minors' nurses, junior doctors and visiting general practitioners. Consultants must know what the reasonable expectations are or the seeds of conflict will be sown.

Health service managers also need to understand the role of the emergency nurse practitioner (ENP). Also, a nurse acting as a practitioner has a defined role which is an enhancement of service for patients. Such ENPs cannot be expected to carry out general nursing, caring and leading, for patients in majors or the resuscitation room. As they say in Yorkshire, 'you gets what you pays for'. This enhanced role for nurses as ENPs – a very productive way of retaining your best nurses – must be reflected in an emergency department's overall nursing staffing levels. Hence why this is also a book for managers.

Having worked alongside our nursing staff as an emergency medicine consultant for 25 years at St Mary's Paddington and for six years at St Charles, Notting Hill (now a nurse-led minor injuries unit), it has been a real joy for me to read this book. The book covers the full range of presentations to 'minors'. It is full of clear medical good sense. Further, this book will help protect all who work in 'minors' from litigation.

Robin Touquet RD FCEM
Emeritus Professor of Emergency Medicine, Imperial College
Locum Consultant, Kingston NHS Trust (including attending Queen Mary's Roehampton MIU)
February 2012

About the author

Mary Dawood RN BSc (Hons) MSc Medical Sociology is a nurse consultant in emergency medicine at Imperial College Healthcare Trust, London. She holds a Postgraduate Diploma in Teaching and Learning in Healthcare and is registered with the Nursing and Midwifery Council (NMC) as a lecturer/practice educator. Prior to her current position, she worked as a lecturer/practitioner where she taught both pre- and post-registration nursing, focusing particularly on the education and training of nurse practitioners. As a nurse consultant, Mary has pursued both an academic and clinical career and has a high profile in emergency nursing in the UK. Her current post as nurse consultant enables her to maintain frequent clinical contact with patients while also supporting and developing the skills of others, in particular supervising Master's students in her specialty. The role also involves research and the strategic development of nursing as a profession. In this capacity she has contributed at policy level to the development of leadership in emergency nursing and was an active member of the Department of Health steering group which implemented and extended non-medical prescribing.

Mary is the Chair of the Emergency Nurse Consultant Association (ENCA) and is the nursing representative on the College of Emergency Medicine Clinical Effectiveness Committee. She is interested in many aspects of emergency care and has published numerous papers on the subject of emergency nursing. She is a co-editor of the recently published *Oxford Handbook of Emergency Nursing*. She is an established speaker, having presented at conferences both nationally and internationally. She is also a member of the editorial board of the health journal *Diversity and Equality in Health and Care* and the *Australasian Journal of Emergency Nursing*. She frequently reviews academic papers for *International Emergency Nursing* (Elsevier), *Emergency Nurse* (RCN Publishing) and *Emergency Medicine Journal* (BMJ Publishing).

Contributors

Bernice Duffy RN
Emergency Nurse Practitioner
The London Hospital
Whitechapel
London

Wendy Martin RN
Senior Sister/Emergency Nurse Practitioner
Emergency Department
Imperial College Healthcare Trust
St Mary's Hospital
London

Lara Ritchie RN BSc (Hons)
Lead Nurse/Emergency Nurse Practitioner
Emergency Department
Imperial College Healthcare Trust
St Mary's Hospital
London

Acknowledgements

The idea for this book was inspired by the many emergency nurse practitioner students I have taught who have frequently asked for a little handbook of tips and prompts to support them in practice. I would like to thank my colleagues Lara Ritchie, Wendy Martin and Bernice Duffy for their valuable contribution to this handbook. I am especially grateful to Mr Robin Touquet, Emeritus Professor of Emergency Medicine at Imperial College Healthcare Trust, for his advice and expert review of the text. Most of all, I thank my husband and family for their unstinting patience and support, without which this handbook could not have come to fruition.

Abbreviations

ABC	airway, breathing, circulation
AC	acromioclavicular
ACL	anterior cruciate ligament
BP	blood pressure
BSA	body surface area
C	cervical
CRP	C-reactive protein
CT	computed tomography
CXR	chest X-ray
DIP	distal interphalangeal
DIPJ	distal interphalangeal joint
DVT	deep venous thrombosis
ECG	electrocardiogram
ED	emergency department
ENP	emergency nurse practitioner
ENT	ear, nose and throat
EP	emergency practitioner
ESR	erythrocyte sedimentation rate
FB	foreign body
FBC	full blood count
GCS	Glasgow Coma Score
GP	general practitioner
GUM	genitourinary medicine
HIV	human immunodeficiency virus
I&D	incision and drainage
IR(ME)R	Ionising Radiation (Medical Exposure) Regulations
ITU	intensive therapy unit
IV	intravenous
LRTI	lower respiratory tract infection
NAI	non-accidental injury
NICE	National Institute for Health and Clinical Excellence
NSAID	non-steroidal anti-inflammatory drug
OPG	orthopantogram

ORIF	open reduction and internal fixation
PGD	Patient Group Directions
PIP	proximal interphalangeal
PIPJ	proximal interphalangeal joint
POM	prescription-only medicine
POP	plaster of Paris
PRN	*pro re nata*
RAPD	relative afferent papillary defect
RICE	rest, ice, compression and elevation
RICER	rest, ice, compression, elevation and rehabilitation
SC	sternoclavicular
SOB	shortness of breath
SUFE	slipped upper femoral epiphysis
TB	tuberculosis
TMT	tarsometatarsal
UCL	ulnar collateral ligament
U&E	urea and electrolytes
URTI	upper respiratory tract infection
UTI	urinary tract infection
VA	visual acuity

Introduction

The development of urgent care centres at the front end of emergency departments and the proliferation of minor injury units and walk-in centres in recent years have led to a parallel rise in emergency practitioners (EPs) whose professional backgrounds range between nursing, physiotherapy and paramedical sciences, with nurses being the predominant group. General practitioners also increasingly work in emergency/urgent care settings, as do Foundation Year 2 doctors.

These hybrid groups of clinicians combine nursing and medical knowledge to deliver timely effective care to patients presenting with a wide range of injuries and illness. The development of these roles has enhanced the quality and completeness of care delivered to patients. EPs in the UK, particularly nurses, are increasingly achieving Master's level education and are in a unique and privileged position to demonstrate the value and effectiveness of advanced nursing practice. All EPs, whatever their professional background, have a duty of care and a responsibility to practise safely and must only carry out procedures that they have been trained for and are competent and confident in executing. As emergency practitioners, they must continue to develop professionally, keep abreast of national guidelines and seek to model their practice and decision making on best available evidence.

In day-to-day practice, EPs see patients with many different presenting complaints and conditions. They are expected to assess, diagnose, treat safely and discharge or refer the patient appropriately. This handbook has been written as an *aide mémoire* to support EPs when they need it most in the clinical setting. It has been written by practising emergency nurse practitioners who understand the thought processes of the EP and the complexities of clinical decision making, particularly for those employed in isolated nurse-led units or those working in the pressurised environment of the emergency department.

The handbook offers straightforward practical advice, highlighting the 'red flags' of specific presentations to prompt extra caution. Whilst it does not describe anatomy or physiology as it assumes this knowledge, it offers reminders of signs which must be considered by the practitioner. Similarly, it assumes that practitioners using this handbook will have well-developed skills such as plastering, suturing and incision and drainage of abscesses.

The layout of each chapter is intended to reflect the thinking processes of the EP, following the 'look, feel, move' method which encourages a uniform approach to assessment and documentation. It encourages health promotion in each patient encounter. It is hoped that this handbook will become the safety companion not just for novice emergency practitioners but also for the more experienced EPs facing busy shifts and undifferentiated patient presentations.

SECTION 1
General issues

CHAPTER 1

Practice advice for the emergency practitioner

GOLDEN RULES AND TIPS FOR BEST PRACTICE

- Remember, patient safety is paramount.
- Always introduce yourself and explain that you are an emergency nurse practitioner (ENP)/general practitioner (GP)/emergency practitioner (EP).
- Ensure your name badge is visible.
- Make pain relief your priority and offer analgesia prior to examination.
- Don't forget to wash your hands and be 'bare below the elbow'.
- Occasionally patients may request to see a doctor; this is usually because they do not understand the role and expertise of the ENP/EP. It is usually sufficient to explain your role.
- Do not become defensive if a patient prefers to see a doctor.
- Try to do your very best for each patient.
- Do not rush either the consultation or your documentation.
- Remember, your documentation is your only defence and you may have to rely on these notes at a later date in court. Make sure they are complete and comprehensive. Draw diagrams wherever you can and particularly in describing injuries attributable to alleged assault.
- By and large, patients want to be a partner in their own care so involve them.
- Ensure privacy and dignity for all your patients appropriate to their presenting problem.
- Assess each patient thoroughly, be fair and objective in your approach.
- Bear in mind that you rarely know the whole story so don't make assumptions or jump to conclusions. Keep an open mind.
- In the case of regular attenders, do not allow the patient's past behaviours to influence your assessment or govern your thinking.
- Don't ignore your 'gut feeling' even if it has no scientific basis.
- Do not be influenced by the assumptions and judgements of others – draw your own conclusions.

- Reassure the patient that X-rays are reviewed by a consultant and that you would contact them if the radiological report recommended a different management plan. Explain that this is a safety mechanism and the need to recall patients is rare.
- Never dismiss the patient's anxiety; if the patient does not seem satisfied with your assessment, ask them what is worrying them most. What may seem trivial and commonplace to you may well be terrifying for the patient.
- Patients understandably fear malignancy but are embarrassed to voice such fears and often need you to articulate that fear and reassure them.
- If the patient does not appear happy with your diagnosis and plan of treatment, ask a colleague to review the patient,
- If the patient does not speak reasonable English, get an interpreter; resist the temptation to just muddle through.
- Avoid using family members to interpret, especially if you are suspicious about the injury.
- Have a chaperone for intimate examinations.
- Always ask about the social circumstances of the patient; it may affect your management.
- Consider referral to occupational therapy/social services if you have any concerns about the ability of older patients to manage at home.
- Remember, domestic violence is prevalent at all levels of society. Do not be afraid to voice your concerns; the patient may be depending on you to recognise the clues.
- Consider non-accidental injury (NAI), including elder abuse, where history and presentation are inconsistent with injury
- Never admonish patients for attending the emergency department (ED) or for calling an ambulance. Deal with the presenting complaint in a professional way and then advise them appropriately.
- Remember alcohol misuse as a cause of falls, collapse, head injury and assault. The patient may have alcohol amnesia or have been unable to attend at the time of injury due to intoxication.
- Use every opportunity to promote health and screen for illness, particularly for problems such as falls and alcohol abuse, for which brief interventions may be helpful.

CHAPTER 2

Avoiding pitfalls and practising safely

'Pitfalls are the bad things that happen to good people'

- The patient understands their complaint better than you do so listen to them.
- Don't become defensive if a patient questions your diagnosis – explain why you think the way you do.
- Don't rush patient assessment or writing notes; this is the surest way to make a mistake or miss something important.
- Always check the patient's identity before administering medications.
- Always read over and sign your notes before closing the episode.
- Don't ignore your intuition even if it has no scientific basis.
- Don't allow your negative feelings or dislike of a patient to affect your objectivity.
- If a patient is being difficult, spend more time with them and try to reassure them.
- If you feel you cannot effectively manage the situation, ask a colleague to help you.
- Listen to your junior colleagues – they may offer valuable insights into the patient's presentation.
- Wherever possible, give written instructions to the patient.
- Ensure that adequate follow-up arrangements are made for the patient but reassure the patient that they can return if they are still worried.

CHAPTER 3

Prescribing

Emergency nurse practitioners are increasingly being registered with the Nursing and Midwifery Council as non-medical prescribers, making this one of the most dramatic developments to have taken place in nursing. There are now approximately 40 000 nurses in the UK qualified to prescribe, and developments continue. The establishment of non-medical prescribing has not only ensured timely treatment for patients; it has also greatly enhanced the autonomy of nurse practitioners working in EDs and urgent care settings.

Nurse practitioners who are not registered as prescribers may use Patient Group Directions (PGD). In practice, this means that a PGD, signed by a doctor and agreed by a pharmacist, can act as a direction to a nurse to supply and/or administer prescription-only medicines (POMs) to patients following their own assessment of patient need. It is, however, preferable for ENPs to become qualified as prescribers to enhance their autonomy and to improve patient safety.

Further useful information in relation to all aspects of prescribing, including legal mechanisms for prescribing, supply and administration of medicines, can be found at the NHS National Prescribing Centre at www.npc.co.uk/prescribers/nmp.htm and at www.nurseprescribing.com.

CHAPTER 4

X-rays and Ionising Radiation (Medical Exposure) Regulations

The EP must be fully aware of the 2000 Ionising Radiation (Medical Exposure) Regulations (IR(ME)R) which came into force on 13 May 2000, replacing the previous regulations known as POPUMET. Most EP education programmes incorporate teaching sessions on the IR(ME)R but EPs also have a personal responsibility to ensure they are competent in this area of practice, which concerns the protection of persons undergoing medical exposure. The IR(ME)R apply to any clinician requesting X-rays.

Different hospitals have different local regulations but a signed request or a password-protected electronic request is always required. The request must be clear and legible and provide the following information:

- unique patient identification
- sufficient details of the medical problem to enable the practitioner to justify the exposure and the operator to verify it against local guidelines, e.g. focus on the mechanism of injury and the clinical diagnosis
- last menstrual period if pregnancy is a possibility
- signature identifying the requester.

The IR(ME)R referrer (the EP) is responsible for providing the medical reasons for the examination being requested. Remember, precise clinical details on the request form assist the radiologist in accurately reporting the X-ray.

The IR(ME)R practitioner (radiographer) is responsible for justifying the exposure, taking into account the potential risks to the patient, the expected benefits, and whether an examination using less ionising radiation would deliver the same clinical information.

X-RAY INTERPRETATION GOLDEN RULES

- Treat the patient, not the radiograph.
- Take a history and examine the patient before requesting a radiograph.

- Request a radiograph only when necessary.
- Never look at a radiograph without seeing the patient and never see the patient without then looking at the radiograph.
- Look at every radiograph, the whole radiograph and the radiograph as a whole.
- Re-examine the patient when there is an incongruity between the radiograph and the expected findings.
- Remember the rule of twos (two views, two joints, two sides, two occasions, two radiographs).
- Take a radiograph before and after a procedure.
- If a radiograph does not look quite right, ask and listen; there is probably something wrong.
- Ensure you are protected by fail-safe mechanisms.

Further reading

Chan O, Touquet R. General principles: how to interpret radiographs. In: Chan O, editor. *ABC of Emergency Radiology*. 2nd ed. London: BMJ Books/Blackwell Publishing; 2007.

Touquet R, Driscoll P, Nicholson D. Teaching in accident and emergency medicine: 10 commandments of accident and emergency radiology. *BMJ*. 1995; **310**: 642–5.

CHAPTER 5

Documentation

!

When writing notes, remember that the Data Protection Act 1998 and Access to Medical Records Act 1990 allow the patient access to their medical records so avoid making judgements, speculations or what might be perceived as pejorative comments. Be impartial and objective and record only facts and observations.

The need for detailed, careful records cannot be overemphasised and they are a crucial component of autonomous practice. It is essential to remember that in most cases, you may be the only clinician to assess the patient and as such, your notes will be the only record of that encounter so make sure they are comprehensive and legible. Remember, you may be called months or sometimes years later to give evidence in court and your notes will be all you can rely on as you are only likely to remember the patient and their injuries in exceptional circumstances.

Remember also that your notes may be perceived as a reflection of you and your practice. Complete, tidy and comprehensive medical records will be to your advantage in any legal case whereas incomplete, untidy or illegible notes will greatly frustrate legal experts and may result in your trust's defence having to settle because your notes could not be counted as legible evidence.

NOTES ON SAFE DOCUMENTATION

- Always use black ink as blue ink does not photocopy well.
- Write your name, date and time of consultation.
- Record the source of the history – patient /paramedic/friend /family/ interpreter.
- Record assault as 'alleged assault'.

- Use diagrams or preprinted anatomical maps to illustrate injuries as well as concise narrative description.
- If electronic records have no facility to draw maps, there is even greater need for precise and detailed anatomical descriptors.
- Record site/side of injury and dominant hand.
- Avoid abbreviations.
- Record the occupation/social history.
- Record positive as well as negative findings, particularly where a negative finding is a relevant exclusionary factor for some conditions.
- When referring a patient to another clinician, document the time of referral and the name of the receiving clinician.
- When seeking an opinion or telephone advice from another clinician, document the name of the clinician giving the advice.
- Ensure your consultations are followed up with a letter to the patient's GP.
- Always sign your record (use of a name stamp enhances professional presentation and ensures greater clarity).

Further reading

Powers M, Barton A, Harris N. *Clinical Negligence*. Haywards Heath, Sussex: Tottel Publishing; 2008.

CHAPTER 6

Police statements

- Police statements may be requested from you from time to time with respect to a patient you may have assessed and treated. This request will be made formally in writing and with the patient's consent.
- Do not give medical/confidential information to the police without the patient's consent.
- Statements should be written carefully and with due diligence.
- Write your statement in a quiet place where you can concentrate. If you have never done this before, ask to see a sample copy from a consultant colleague.
- Make sure you have the patient's notes to hand and keep your statement concise and to the point.
- State only the facts and provide explanation in lay terms for any medical terms you may have to use.
- Do not give your opinion on possible cause or outcome.
- State any investigations and treatment you gave. In the case of lacerations, state the size and depth of the wound and how many stitches you inserted to close the wound.
- Read through it before signing and dating each page.
- Your signature should be witnessed by another party.
- Complete the form to claim the statement writing fee.
- Keep a copy of the statement in case you are requested to attend court.

CHAPTER 7

Paediatric considerations

Children make up 25–30% of attendances in many EDs in the UK and many more attend minor injury units and walk-in centres. Most EDs now have specialist paediatric staff but this may not be the case with minor injury or walk-in centres where practitioners will still be expected to safely manage or refer children who present with minor injury or illness.

Despite the fact that children make up a significant number of attendees, few nurse practitioner training programmes have specific paediatric content and most EPs do not have paediatric training. Therefore, EPs working in stand-alone minor injury units or walk-in centres have a professional responsibility to ensure they have at the very minimum basic paediatric life support skills and a fundamental understanding of normal paediatric physiological values and milestones.

Children are different from adults anatomically, physiologically and emotionally. Because of their size, they are more vulnerable to injury and their injuries may be more complex than those sustained by adults.

In assessing an unwell child, it is essential to know and consider normal paediatric physiological parameters.

Table 7.1 Normal expected childhood values

Age	*Respiratory rate*	*Heart rate*	*Systolic blood pressure*
<1	30–40	110–160	70–90
1–2	25–35	100–150	80–95
2–5	25–30	95–140	80–100
5–12	20–25	80–120	90–110
>12	15–20	60–100	100–120

DEALING WITH PARENTS

Parents will be worried and upset if their child is injured or unwell. It is essential to behave in a calm and competent way, offering reassurance. Be sensitive to their anxiety and keep them consistently informed about what is happening. Involve them as much as possible with care and avoid separating them from their child at any point as this only adds to both the child's and parents' distress. Relieving pain is a key priority.

SECTION 2
Musculoskeletal

CHAPTER 8

Assault

Assault is a common reason for patients to attend the ED or urgent care setting, so EPs need to be familiar with the process of assessing and documenting injuries associated with alleged assault.

Most importantly, you may be asked to provide a police statement or even attend court at a much later date so it is absolutely imperative that you examine the patient thoroughly and document every finding, however trivial it may seem to be at the time.

SAFETY TIPS

- Each assault is an alleged assault.
- Always use diagrams; if this is not possible because of the software in use, there is even greater need to be detailed and meticulous in your description of injuries.
- Some patients may deny assault, particularly in situations such as domestic violence.
- Be aware that domestic abuse is prevalent in all social classes and ethnic groups and in some societies it is not considered to be a criminal offence.
- Remember domestic violence affects men as well as women.
- If you suspect domestic violence as the cause of injury, ask whether there are children involved.
- If children are involved in any way, this is a safeguarding issue so act to protect the children as well as your patient.
- Remember that abuse of the elderly and vulnerable adults is a sad reality and increasingly common. Follow local safeguarding guidelines.
- In recent years there has been a worrying increase in the abuse of hired home helps, amounting in some cases to 'modern-day slavery'. Be vigilant, particularly where the patient does not speak English and is brought in by the employer with injuries that are not consistent with the history. In such situations, always get an interpreter and insist on seeing the patient without the employer in the room.

- Many patients alleging assault may also be under the influence of alcohol but never assume that fluctuating or deteriorating conscious level is due to alcohol. If concerned, get help.
- If the patient has a number of injuries, be methodical and assess each one in turn.
- Document where the alleged assault took place and if any implement was used.
- In assessing lacerations, use the '5 Ss': Site, Size/shape, Sharp/blunt, Sterile/clean or dirty wound, Structures (deep structures, vessels, tendons, nerves, bones).
- Only request imaging or investigations essential to diagnoses.
- Consider the need for tetanus immunisation or treatment for human bites. Be aware of possible penetration of the metacarpophalangeal (knuckle) joint, e.g. by a tooth.
- Document in detail any treatment given and follow-up care arranged.
- If assault is due to domestic abuse, encourage the patient to report it if they have not already done so. If they cannot be encouraged to report the incident, give them information about how to get help if they change their mind. Make sure they do not leave the department on their own.
- If the patient has children, follow local safeguarding policies, ensuring appropriate professionals/agencies are involved to protect the children.

CHAPTER 9

Head injury

Simple head injury with or without skin trauma is a common presentation in the ED, with only a very small minority being classified as severe. Careful detailed history taking is essential as assessment is not always straightforward and subtleties can be missed. EPs are advised to act with caution and ask for help if they are unsure or the presenting signs are ambiguous.

Many patients who present with a simple head injury do so days after the event and are concerned by persistent symptoms. Most patients will be discharged with head injury instructions but for the few who have sustained a more serious injury, the signs may be less than obvious so meticulous assessment is essential. **Follow NICE guidelines.**

- Always consider the possibility of cervical (C)-spine injury in any head injury.
- Never assume that a patient is 'drunk' where there is altered conscious level/Glasgow Coma Score (GCS).
- Don't forget ABCs and refer to a doctor if there is a history of loss of consciousness.
- Remember, patients on anticoagulants and aspirin are more vulnerable to intracerebral haemorrhage.
- Children can sustain significant intracranial injury from shaking without visible skull/scalp injury.
- Be aware of odontoid fractures in the elderly.

HISTORY

- Indicate source of history if not the patient.
- Mechanism of injury.
- Time of injury.
- Witnessed loss of consciousness.
- Ongoing amnesia.

- Headache not relieved with analgesia.
- Nausea/vomiting/frequency of vomiting.
- Visual disturbance.
- Giddiness/balance disturbance.
- Amnesia before and/or after event.
- Speech or articulation disturbance (this may be very subtle, not apparent to the assessor and only noticed by the patient or family).
- Poor concentration.
- Persistent drowsiness.
- Any fitting.

PAST MEDICAL HISTORY

- Any bleeding disorder is relevant.
- Previous neurological illness.
- Medication history (on anticoagulant).
- Known allergy.
- Social history/occupation is relevant (especially where driving or handling machinery is involved).

EXAMINATION

- Observe and document any obvious signs:
  - abnormal/unsteady gait
  - check pupils and eye movements
  - lacerations/abrasions to face/head
  - look for associated injuries, especially neck
  - bilateral periorbital haematoma (panda eyes), bruising in the mastoid area, blood in the auditory meatus (signs of basal skull fracture).
- Assess GCS – if less than 12, get help.
- Check vital signs, including pulse, blood pressure (BP) and respiration rate, and document them.
- Feel scalp for tenderness, swelling or bruising and palpate any open wound for a fracture.
- Assess power in limbs/reflexes.
- Assess cranial nerves.

Table 9.1 Cranial nerves

Nerve	*Classification*	*Major functions*	*Assessment*
I Olfactory	Sensory	Smell	Identify a familiar scent with eyes closed
II Optic	Sensory	Vision (acuity and field of vision); pupil reactivity to light and accommodation	Identify the number of fingers you're holding up in each of four visual quadrants
III Oculomotor	Motor	Eyelid elevation; pupil size and reactivity	Check pupillary responses by shining a bright light on one pupil; both pupils should constrict. To check accommodation, move your finger toward the patient's nose; the pupils should constrict and converge. Ask patient to look up, down, laterally and diagonally
IV Trochlear	Motor	Extrinsic ocular muscles (turn eye downward and laterally)	Have patient look down and in
V Trigeminal	Both	Chewing; facial and mouth sensation; corneal reflex (sensory)	Ask patient to hold the mouth open while you try to close it and to move the jaw laterally against your hand. With patient's eyes closed, touch her face with cotton and have her identify the area touched
VI Abducens	Motor	Turns eye laterally	Have patient move the eyes from side to side
VII Facial	Both	Facial expression; taste; corneal reflex (motor); eyelid and lip closure	Ask patient to smile, raise eyebrows, and keep eyes and lips closed while you try to open them
VIII Acoustic	Sensory	Hearing; equilibrium	Use tuning fork or rub your fingers, place a ticking watch or whisper near each ear
IX Glossopharyngeal	Both	Gagging and swallowing (sensory); taste	Touch back of throat with sterile tongue depressor or cotton-tipped applicator. Have patient swallow
X Vagus	Both	Gagging and swallowing (motor); speech (phonation)	Assess gag and swallowing with cranial nerve IX. Assess vocal quality
XI Spinal accessory	Motor	Shoulder movement; head rotation	Have patient shrug shoulders and turn head from side to side
XII Hypoglossal	Motor	Tongue movement; speech (articulation)	Have patient stick out tongue and move it internally from cheek to cheek. Assess articulation

MANAGEMENT OF HEAD INJURY

- Follow NICE guidelines and consider the need for computed tomography (CT) to exclude cerebral bleed.
- Refer for medical assessment if evidence of:
  - altered conscious level
  - alcohol involved
  - severe headache not relieved with simple analgesia
  - persistent vomiting
  - neurological signs/symptoms
  - amnesia.
- The patient can be discharged if they remain alert with no significant injury but postconcussion symptoms; can go home with a responsible adult who must be vigilant for the following 24–36 hours.

> IMPORTANT
>
> Give the patient written head injury instructions but also go through the instructions with the patient and carer so they fully understand what to expect and what signs or symptoms are potentially more serious. Offer reassurance but also be realistic and advise the patient that vague symptoms may endure for a good few weeks.

SCALP LACERATION

- Ensure sufficient analgesia/anaesthesia.
- Clean thoroughly and debride if needed.
- Palpate for fracture before suturing.
- Use 3/0 suture for scalp.
- As far as possible, wash blood out of patient's hair. If needed, shave hair by scalp wound but never shave eyebrows.
- Use a pressure dressing if the wound is still oozing.
- Immunise against tetanus as indicated.
- Send home with simple analgesia and head injury advice.
- Ensure that there is necessary support for older patients.
- Advise parents/carers on what signs to look out for and when to bring the patient back for further assessment.

CHAPTER 10

Facial/nasal injury

Most isolated facial injuries seen by the EP will be due to sporting injuries or assaults. When assessing injury attributed to assault, be meticulous in your documentation as you may be called upon to write police statements and give evidence in court at a much later date. It is only then that you will appreciate the detail of your documentation.

> Perform a rapid assessment to exclude any evidence of respiratory distress or persistent cough/dyspnoea. Consider C-spine injury. If concerned, get senior help. Consider NAI and especially domestic violence.

HISTORY

- Indicate the source of history, if not the patient.
- Document mechanism of injury to face but also consider injuries to head and neck.
- If alleged assault, brief history including when, where and how.
- Time and date of injury.
- Any loss of consciousness.
- Headache.
- Any dizziness, visual disturbance, nausea, vomiting.
- Speech disturbance.
- Altered facial sensation.
- Epistaxis at time of injury or since.
- Dental injury.

PAST MEDICAL HISTORY

- ?Anticoagulants/aspirin or bleeding disorder.
- Tetanus status.
- Known allergy.

EXAMINATION

Look

- Signs of head injury.
- Obvious swelling, bruising, deformity or loss of symmetry to facial bones.
- Lacerations to face/ears/eyelid/tarsal plate (the plate of strong dense fibrous connective tissue that forms the supporting structure of the eyelid).
- Neurological deficit. Check facial nerves; altered sensation over cheek and lip suggests infraorbital nerve injury and most likely a fracture.
- Subconjunctival haemorrhage, diplopia, restricted eye movements.
- Bite occlusion.
- Check for septal deviation and septal haematoma (the latter can result in septal perforation if not drained).
- Check for loose or missing teeth.

Feel

- Feel for clinical features of fractures.
- Feel for tenderness in facial bones.
- Palpate for step deformity on orbital margin and zygomatic prominence.
- Feel for crepitus due to air from maxillary sinus.

INVESTIGATIONS

- Do a full set of neurological observations.
- Check temperature if late presentation.
- Always check visual acuity (VA); facial fracture can cause orbital haematoma and optic nerve compression.

X-RAYS

- If you suspect a fracture to the mandible, ask for an orthopantogram (OPG) view. The mandible is a ring-like structure which is predisposed to multiple fractures (the pretzel rule). Once a single mandibular fracture is identified, it is essential that an accompanying fracture on the contralateral side is excluded.

- If you suspect a maxillary/zygoma fracture, ask for facial views.The inferior orbital rim is a common location for displaced and comminuted fractures. These injuries can be isolated but they are often associated with orbital floor fractures.
- The walls of the maxillary antrum, fluid level or opaque antrum, tear drop sign (indicates blow-out fracture).
- Routine nasal X-ray is not usually indicated.

Facial X-rays can be difficult to interpret accurately so get help if unsure.

MANAGEMENT OF FACIAL FRACTURES

- Discuss all facial fractures with the ED consultant or maxillofacial team.
- Patients with visual symptoms, numbness/altered sensation, altered bite, displaced fracture or blow-out fracture will need immediate assessment by specialty consultants and antibiotic cover.
- Uncomplicated fractures can be sent to the maxillofacial clinic but ensure antibiotic cover.
- Isolated dental problems such as very loose or chipped teeth can be referred to the patient's own dentist.

MANAGEMENT OF FACIAL LACERATIONS

- Refer complex facial lacerations to the maxillofacial team.
- Eyelid laceration/tarsal plate involvement should be referred to the ophthalmologists for closure.
- Steri-Strips or glue may be sufficient to close superficial facial wounds.
- Only consider suturing facial wounds if competent and confident to do so, particularly in relation to the vermilion border of the lip or the eyebrow where, if not undertaken skilfully, it will leave an unsightly scar.
- Ensure laceration is thoroughly cleansed and debrided if necessary before suturing.
- Use 3/0 sutures for the scalp and 5/0 for the face.
- Always be honest with the patient and advise about scarring, particularly the likelihood of keloid scars.

ANIMAL/HUMAN BITES TO THE FACE

- Ensure good analgesia.
- Clean thoroughly.
- Cover wounds with saline soaks.
- Ensure tetanus cover and tetanus immunoglobulin as necessary.
- Provide antibiotic cover and refer to maxillofacial surgeons.

EAR LACERATIONS

- Examine and exclude injury to the ear canal.
- Cartilage has poor healing qualities and lacerations to the pinna or tragus may be easier to glue than to suture.
- Continuous bleeding will need a pressure bandage to prevent haematoma formation.
- If an earlobe haematoma develops, it will need drainage to prevent cartilage destruction.

CHAPTER 11

Neck pain

A history of trauma with cervical spine tenderness and abnormal neurological signs warrants immediate immobilisation in a hard collar, head blocks and referral for medical assessment.

ACUTE TORTICOLLIS

Most patients presenting to the ED with acute neck pain/spasm have torticollis but it is important to keep an open mind and exclude trauma or infection as causative factors.

Torticollis, sometimes referred to as 'wryneck', is caused by involuntary contractions of the neck muscles. Acute torticollis usually develops overnight and results in painful, palpable neck spasms the following morning. Symptoms usually resolve spontaneously within a few days.

CAUTION

Torticollis can present as a dystonic reaction secondary to medications such as phenothiazines, metoclopramide, haloperidol, carbamazepine and phenytoin.

IMMEDIATE CHECK

Exclude trauma, cervical spine tenderness or neurological deficit. Cervical spine injury is unlikely if the patient has no neck pain or tenderness, no neurological signs or symptoms, no loss of consciousness, normal mental status and no distracting injury.

Initial actions

- Document:
  - history of complaint
  - past medical history
  - medications
  - allergies
  - social history.
- If no trauma, exclude neurological signs and symptoms.
- **Abnormal neurological signs must be referred to a doctor (middle grade or above).**
- Ensure that the patient is systemically well; exclude pyrexia.
- Advise the patient on analgesia.
- Advise on exercises.
- Refer to a physiotherapist with caution. Physiotherapy needs to be started immediately to be beneficial.
- Also consider the potential risks of overmedicalising the condition as the patient may delay commencing exercises until review by physiotherapy.

TRAUMATIC NECK SPRAIN

Avoid the term 'whiplash' as it can have legal ramifications.

Traumatic neck sprain usually occurs when a stationary or slowly moving vehicle is hit from behind, forcing the occupants' necks into extreme extension and often compression (due to impact with the ceiling of the car) and then flexion (as the car decelerates).

Signs and symptoms

There is often no pain at the time of the incident. Pain and neck discomfort may take a few hours to develop and are usually worse the next day. The pain is normally worse in the paravertebral cervical spine area. There may be difficulty turning the neck from side to side and tenderness in the shoulders or down the arms. The patient may complain of headaches, dizziness and poor concentration.

Management

- Verbal advice and positive reassurance about prognosis are important and should be supplemented with written advice.
- Regular analgesia and non-steroidal anti-inflammatory drugs (NSAIDs) are usually recommended.

- The patient should be encouraged to mobilise. An advice sheet with exercises that can be undertaken at home may be given to the patient.
- Soft collars are not usually recommended.
- Physiotherapy should be instituted if suspicious of osteoarthritis in the cervical spine and symptoms persist.

CHAPTER 12

Chest

Common presentations include fractures and/or bruising to ribs.

IMMEDIATE CHECK

- Ensure the patient has no difficulty in breathing and check vital signs, especially heart rate, respiration rate and oxygen saturation.
- Get help if there are any signs of difficulty in breathing.
- Patients presenting with a chest wall injury and associated respiratory or cardiac problems should be assessed by a doctor.

FLAIL CHEST

!

Flail chest is an instability of the chest wall due to multiple rib fractures, or detachment of the sternum from the ribs as a result of a severe chest injury. The loose chest segment moves in a direction which is the reverse of normal; that is, the segment moves inward during inspiration and outward during expiration (paradoxical respiration). Other signs include shortness of breath, cyanosis and extreme pain in the area of trauma.

HISTORY

- Describe mechanism of injury (low-velocity injury is likely to cause injury to chest wall only).
- Patients will usually present in pain which is worse on inspiration or springing the chest).
- If no history of injury, consider cardiac/respiratory cause of pain.
- Date and time of injury.

- Character, site and onset of pain.
- Pain worse on movement.
- Any breathlessness at rest.
- Occupation.
- Relevant past medical history.
- Current medications.
- Allergies.

EXAMINATION

- Undress the patient.
- Observe general perfusion and respiratory rate.
- Check skin integrity, looking for bruising, laceration, abrasion and scars.
- Observe chest movement; listen for equal air entry and percuss bilaterally.
- Chest X-ray is not necessary to diagnose associated rib fracture but necessary to exclude pneumothorax or underlying injury or contusions.
- If sternal fracture is suspected, request chest X-ray, lateral sternal X-ray and electrocardiogram (ECG), and refer to a doctor.

UNCOMPLICATED SUSPECTED RIB FRACTURES

- Ensure patient has adequate analgesia.
- Advise regular deep breathing exercises to avoid chest infection.
- Advise patient to return if breathing problems develop.
- Vital signs should be recorded as normal on discharge.
- Ensure that elderly patients with minor chest injury can cope at home.
- Consider occupational therapy referral prior to discharge.

CHAPTER 13

Back pain

Back pain is a very common presentation and affects most people at some point during their life. Most cases of back pain are not serious; they are often the result of heavy lifting and are associated with pain and stiffness in the lower back.

TYPES OF BACK PAIN

- *Specific back pain* – pain that is associated with an underlying health condition or damage to the spine.
- *Non-specific back pain* – where the pain is not caused by serious damage or disease but by sprains, muscle strains, minor injuries or a pinched or irritated nerve.

CAUTION

Bowel and bladder disturbance suggests cauda equina syndrome. This syndrome may require emergency surgery to avoid permanent damage to bowel and bladder control or even paralysis.

Patients with any of the following symptoms need referral for a full medical assessment.

- Presentation under age 20 or onset over the age of 55.
- Violent trauma, i.e. fall from a height, road traffic accident.
- Constant, progressive, non-mechanical pain.
- Systemically unwell.
- Weight loss.
- Drug abuse, positive HIV status
- Persisting severe restriction of lumbar flexion.
- Widespread neurological signs and symptoms.

SIMPLE BACKACHE

- Often results from heavy lifting.
- Presentation between ages 20 and 55.
- Usually lumbosacral region.
- No tenderness in spinous process.
- Pain is 'mechanical' in nature.
- Varies with physical activity and with time.
- Patient generally otherwise well.
- Recovery: 90% in 4–6 weeks.
- Attributed to muscle or ligamentous strain or injury.
- Can be caused by nerve root pain (nerve from spinal cord is irritated or compressed).
- Pain can vary from mild to severe.

Patients with the following symptoms need referral for a full medical assessment.

- Unilateral leg/thigh pain worse than low back pain.
- Pain generally radiates to foot or toes.
- Numbness and paraesthesia in the same distribution.
- Nerve irritation signs.
- Reduced straight-leg raise which reproduces back pain (detects tension on L5/S1 nerve root).
- Motor, sensory or reflex change.

MANAGEMENT OF SIMPLE BACK PAIN

- If no 'red flags', reassure and give positive information on prognosis.
- Encourage early activity: give exercise information sheets and advice leaflets.
- Give education on the nature of back pain and address psychosocial features and prognostic importance.
- Provide NSAIDs and simple analgesia.
- Muscle relaxants such as diazepam may be useful if back muscles are tense.
- Refer for early physiotherapy but only for a new attack, not for recurrent or chronic back pain.

CHAPTER 14

Shoulder injury

COMMON PRESENTATIONS

- Shoulder dislocation.
- Fractured clavicle.
- Fractured neck of humerus.
- Rotator cuff injuries.
- Abnormal calcification.

> **IMMEDIATE CHECK**
>
> - Severe pain.
> - Obvious deformity/numbness over deltoid.
> - Neurovascular deficit in the arm.

Remember, a fall onto the outstretched hand may also cause fractures to the radius and clavicle and supracondylar fractures to the humerus. Don't forget that shoulder pain may be referred pain from the neck.

HISTORY

- Describe the mechanism of injury (consider posterior dislocation if injury sustained during an epileptic fit).
- Site/side.
- Dominant hand.
- Occupation.
- Past medical history.
- Current medications (anticonvulsants may be relevant as posterior dislocation of the shoulder may be caused by an epileptic seizure).
- Allergies.

EXAMINATION

Look

- Obvious deformity.
- A visible step over the acromioclavicular joint may indicate injury.
- Flattening of shoulder and prominence of the acromioclavicular joint may indicate dislocation of the shoulder.
- Swelling, lacerations, wounds, bruising and erythema.
- Local swelling and tenderness in the front of the shoulder (consider impingement).
- Winging of scapula (a winging scapula is associated with damage or a contusion to the long thoracic nerve of the shoulder and/or weakness in the serratus anterior muscle).

Feel

- Temperature of skin (compare with unaffected side).
- If there is sensation/numbness over the deltoid, check:
  - chest wall
  - anterior glenohumeral joint and coracoid process
  - bony tenderness of clavicle, scapula, acromioclavicular joint, head and neck of humerus
  - acromioclavicular and sternoclavicular joints.
- Check the biceps tendon.
- Check cervical spine.

Move

- Check all movements (abduction, adduction, internal/external rotation and circumduction).
- Localised tenderness under acromion, inability to initiate shoulder abduction and painful arc (rotator cuff tear).
- Pain on resisted abduction (supraspinatus tendonitis).
- Pain on resisted internal rotation (subscapularis tendonitis).
- Pain on resisted external rotation (infraspinatus disease).

IMPORTANT

The joints above and below (neck and elbow) should also be examined to exclude the likelihood of referred shoulder pain from other pathology.

INVESTIGATIONS

- X-ray if obvious deformity or bony tenderness.
- In interpreting shoulder X-rays, always ensure a good lateral view.

MANAGEMENT

Dislocated shoulder

- Urgent X-ray, then reduction.
- Give analgesia before X-ray.
- Important: check neurovascular status before and after reduction.
- Reduction by ED team with sedation and analgesia.
- Apply collar and cuff.
- Follow-up in fracture clinic.

Rotator cuff injury

In the young person, tears to the rotator cuff sometimes occur with a sudden overhead movement of the arm. The patient may describe a sudden tearing sensation followed by severe pain shooting from the upper shoulder area, both anterior and posterior and towards the elbow. Loss of active abduction but retained passive abduction is suggestive of an acute rotator cuff tear. Loss of abduction and significant pain and loss of muscle power are suggestive of a large tear.

These patients need referral to orthopaedics.

Chronic rotator cuff tear

- May be more common in the older person.
- Pain usually is worse at night and may interfere with sleep.
- Gradual weakness and decreased shoulder motion develop as the pain worsens.
- Exclude bony injury and refer to physiotherapy for ongoing management.

Fractured clavicle

Refer to orthopaedics if the skin is tented, there is neurovascular injury or a comminuted fracture close to the acromioclavicular (AC) or sternoclavicular (SC) joint.

Acromioclavicular joint injury

These injuries are common, especially in contact sports and car accidents. The AC joint is located at the top of the shoulder where the acromion process and the clavicle meet. Torn ligaments and separation of the AC joint can occur, depending on the force and mechanism of injury.

If the AC joint is tender but there is no step, use a broad arm sling. If the X-ray shows AC joint separation, refer to orthopaedics.

Sternoclavicular joint injury

This is not a common injury. Symptoms include pain and swelling and dimpling of the skin over the SC joint.

> Be aware that patients with severe SC injury can have difficulty breathing, painful swallowing and abnormal pulses caused by compression of the trachea, oesophagus and blood vessels.

Simple sprains to the SC joint are treated with a sling and anti-inflammatory medications. Refer to orthopaedics if manipulation is required.

Neck of humerus

Displaced

- U-slab or hanging cast, otherwise collar and cuff. Refer to fracture clinic.
- Ensure good analgesia is provided.
- As these patients are often female and elderly, consider the need for social support.

Abnormal calcification

- Patient may present with acute severe pain over the shoulder with loss of movement.
- X-ray may show fluffy calcification over the subacromial area.
- Treat with NSAIDs if not contraindicated.
- Fit a sling.
- Refer to review clinic or GP for further management.

Sprain/soft tissue injury

- Encourage early mobilisation. Provide pain relief and advice on exercises.
- Fit a broad arm sling.
- Provide analgesia and consider NSAIDs.
- If there is significant loss of function, refer for follow-up to review clinic/GP.

Remember that, in most cases, the enemy of shoulder joint recovery is immobility.

CHAPTER 15

Upper arm injuries

COMMON PRESENTATIONS

➤ Fracture of the shaft of humerus.
➤ Ruptured head of biceps.

Remember, as with all limb injuries, the joint above and the joint below should be checked.

IMMEDIATE CHECK

➤ Pain.
➤ Pallor.
➤ Pulselessness.
➤ Paraesthesia.
➤ Paralysis.

HISTORY

➤ Describe mechanism of injury.
➤ Onset/duration of symptoms.
➤ Site/side.
➤ Dominant hand.
➤ Occupation and hobbies.
➤ Social history.
➤ Relevant past medical history.
➤ Current medications.
➤ Allergies.

EXAMINATION

Look

- Obvious deformity.
- 'Popeye' sign in cases of ruptured long head of biceps.
- Swelling.
- Bruising (extensive bruising of the upper arm is usually indicative of a fracture).
- Erythema.
- Wounds.

Feel

- Sensation over deltoid and radial nerve.
- Bony tenderness over clavicle, scapula, acromioclavicular joint, head, neck and shaft of humerus, elbow.
- Check biceps tendon.

Move

- Shoulder movements (see Chapter 14).
- Elbow movements (see Chapter 16).
- Fractures to the neck and shaft of humerus are more common in older women due to osteoporosis.

INVESTIGATIONS

- X-ray in cases of suspected fracture of the shaft of humerus.
- Consider X-ray of the elbow in cases of ruptured biceps to exclude avulsion fracture where the biceps inserts into the radial tuberosity.

MANAGEMENT

Fracture of the shaft of humerus

- Analgesia.
- If non-displaced, manage in collar and cuff.
- Fracture clinic follow-up.
- If displaced or any neurological deficit, refer to on-call orthopaedic team.

CAUTION

As these injuries are more common in older patients, occupational therapist involvement should be considered, as should referral to the falls clinic in line with local policy.

These types of injury have also been linked to elder abuse and this should be considered when taking the history and examining the patient.

Ruptured long head of biceps

- Often strength is maintained as the biceps has two heads.
- In incomplete ruptures, the management is rest, ice, elevation and physiotherapy.
- In complete ruptures, the patient should be referred to orthopaedic surgeons.

CHAPTER 16

Elbow injury

COMMON PRESENTATIONS

- ➤ Radial head fracture.
- ➤ Olecranon fracture.
- ➤ Olecranon bursitis.
- ➤ Supracondylar fracture (rare in adults, common in children; see Chapter 24).
- ➤ Dislocated elbow (requires significant force).
- ➤ Lateral epicondylitis (tennis elbow).
- ➤ Medial epicondylitis (golfer's elbow, very uncommon).
- ➤ Pulled elbow in a child.

As with all traumatic limb injuries, you must check the joint above and the joint below.

COMMON MISSED INJURIES

Greenstick injuries around wrist, radial head fracture, clavicle fracture, fractured neck of humerus.

> IMMEDIATE CHECK
>
> - ➤ Pain.
> - ➤ Pallor.
> - ➤ Pulselessness.
> - ➤ Paraesthesia.
> - ➤ Paralysis.

HISTORY

- Describe mechanism of injury.
- Onset/duration of symptoms.
- Site/side.
- Dominant hand.
- Occupation and hobbies.
- Social history.
- Relevant past medical history.
- Current medications.
- Allergies.

EXAMINATION

Look

- Obvious deformity.
- Colour of skin.
- Erythema.
- Wounds.
- Bruising.
- Swelling.
- Wasting compared to other limb.

Feel

- Skin temperature.
- Sensation over brachial artery, radial and median nerve distribution.
- Bony tenderness over humeral condyles, olecranon, proximal radius and ulna.

Move

- Flexion.
- Extension.
- Pronation.
- Supination (fracture of forearm bones is unlikely if there is full pronation and supination).

Loss of full extension is suggestive of a fracture to the radial head. The fracture may not be obvious on X-ray but evidence of an effusion (fat pad/sail sign) may indicate a fracture.

MANAGEMENT OF ELBOW INJURIES

Radial head fracture

- Adequate analgesia.
- Collar and cuff.
- Fracture clinic follow-up.
- Consider the need for social support in the older person.

Olecranon fracture

If the articular surface is involved, refer to orthopaedics immediately. Otherwise:

- adequate analgesia
- back-slab and fracture clinic
- broad arm sling
- orthopaedic referral.

Olecranon bursitis

- Adequate analgesia.
- Rest, ice, elevation, NSAIDs.
- Exclude infection – treat with antibiotics if necessary.

Dislocated elbow

- Immobilise on pillows.
- Adequate analgesia, IV usually required.
- Regular neurovascular observations.
- Senior support for reduction.
- Orthopaedic referral.

Supracondylar fracture (rare in adults)

- Adequate analgesia.
- Support limb (pillows or sling as patient comfort dictates).
- Regular neurovascular observations.
- Orthopaedic referral.

Lateral epicondylitis (tennis elbow) and medial epicondylitis (golfer's elbow)

The clue to this diagnosis will be in the history taking. Usually a gradual increase in the severity of symptoms, coupled with activities that strain the elbow (such as tennis and golf).

- Analgesia.
- Rest.
- Avoid overuse activities.
- In some cases, physiotherapy and steroid injections may be required.

CHAPTER 17

Wrist and forearm injury

Wrist injuries are a very common presentation in emergency settings. Fractures of the distal radius and ulna account for three-quarters of wrist injuries. The carpal bones are injured less often but account for up to 10% of injuries to the structures of the hand.

Fall on the outstretched hand – check for Colles' fracture, scaphoid, head of radius, capitellum, supracondyle, humerus, clavicle.

CAUTION

Do not underestimate the impact of wrist fractures; failure to accurately identify or treat can result in substantial morbidity such as chronic pain and limited function. As with all limb injuries, assessment of the joint above and the joint below is imperative to exclude concomitant injury. This is particularly important if the mechanism of injury is one of high energy or force.

COMMON PRESENTATIONS

- Colles' fracture.
- Smith's fracture.
- Scaphoid fracture.
- Fractured shaft of radius and/or ulna.

LESS COMMON PRESENTATIONS

- Monteggia fracture (fracture of the ulna with dislocation of the radial head).
- Galeazzi fracture (fracture of the radius with injury to the distal radio-ulnar joint).

IMMEDIATE CHECK

Particularly important where wrist deformity is apparent. Ensure early analgesia as these injuries can be very distressing and painful.

- Pain.
- Pallor.
- Pulselessness.
- Paraesthesia.
- Paralysis.

HISTORY

- Describe mechanism of injury.
- Onset/duration of symptoms.
- Site/side.
- Dominant hand.
- Occupation and hobbies.
- Social history.
- Relevant past medical history.
- Current medications.
- Allergies.

EXAMINATION

Look

- Obvious deformity.
- Swelling.
- Bruising.
- Wounds.

Feel

- Pulse.
- Sensation (check radial, median and ulna nerves).
- Bony tenderness.

Move

Movement should be kept to a minimum. The arm should be supported either in a broad arm sling or on pillows.

INVESTIGATIONS

X-ray the whole forearm, including wrist and elbow joints (to avoid missing Monteggia and Galeazzi injuries).

WRIST FRACTURES

Undisplaced Colles' fracture

Colles' fracture tends to be the general term applied to describe any fracture of the distal radius, with or without involvement of the ulna, particularly where there is dorsal displacement of the fracture fragment. Nonetheless, a Colles' fracture is specifically a fracture through the distal metaphysis about 2 cm proximal to the articular surface of the radius. These fractures are not always straightforward and can have associated complications, including:

- median nerve impairment
- extensor pollicis longus tendon rupture (long term, not acute)
- stiffness, malunion and chronic pain.

Timely reduction and early orthopaedic involvement are essential to avoid these problems and are indicated in displaced or impacted fractures.

It is essential for the EP to ensure urgent orthopaedic follow-up for those patients with undisplaced fractures not seen at the time of injury by the orthopaedic team.

Management of undisplaced Colles' fracture

Ice, analgesia and a plaster of Paris (POP) back-slab with the wrist in 15° flexion and 15° ulnar deviation is appropriate initial treatment for this group of patients.

- High sling.
- Analgesia.
- Follow-up in fracture clinic.

Displaced Colles' fracture

Appropriately trained EPs can reduce these fractures using a haematoma block. If this is not possible, the patient should be referred to the ED registrar for manipulation.

- Analgesia.
- POP back-slab.
- Broad arm sling.
- Check x-ray post reduction and providing position is acceptable, the patient can be discharged and followed up in the fracture clinic.

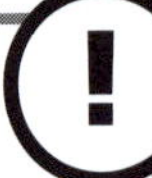

Consider the potential for post-reduction swelling with development of compartment syndrome and advise the patient accordingly.

If the patient is elderly or vulnerable in any sense, consider the need for added social support.

Smith's fracture

A Smith's fracture is an injury to the distal radius with volar displacement of the distal fragment. This is an unstable fracture most commonly caused by falling on to the back of the hand. These patients need immediate referral to orthopaedics for possible open reduction and internal fixation (ORIF) and further management.

Plaster of Paris may be used but needs careful observation to ensure the fracture does not further displace.

Keep the patient nil by mouth until a decision has been made about management.

Shaft of radius and ulna fractures (Monteggia/Galeazzi)

A Monteggia fracture is a fracture of the ulna, with an associated dislocation of the radial head within the elbow joint.

A Galeazzi fracture is a fracture of the radius, with an associated injury of the distal radio-ulnar joint of the wrist.

These are both complicated fractures which need immediate orthopaedic referral, analgesia and immobilisation.

Undisplaced ulna fracture

- Analgesia.
- Above-elbow back-slab.
- Fracture clinic follow-up as per local policy.

Barton's fracture

This is an intra-articular fracture of the dorsal margin of the distal radius which extends into the radiocarpal joint.

Bennett's fracture

This is an intra-articular fracture/dislocation of the base of the first metacarpal where a small fragment of the first metacarpal continues to articulate with the trapezium.

Rolando's fracture

This is a comminuted intra-articular fracture through the base of the thumb.

Treatment for Barton's, Bennett's and Rolando's fractures

The above three fractures are complicated and need immediate referral to orthopaedics for ORIF (see also Chapter 18).

Immobilise the limb and give adequate analgesia.

Fracture to carpal bones (radial aspect)

Scaphoid injury

The scaphoid is the most frequently injured carpal bone, accounting for 60–70% of all carpal fractures. EPs need to remember that failure to assess, X-ray and/or subsequently manage this injury appropriately is a common cause of litigation.

> **SCAPHOID INJURY** !
>
> Scaphoid fractures are sometimes associated with other injuries of the wrist, such as dislocation of the radiocarpal joint. Consider a scaphoid injury where there is:
>
> - tenderness in the anatomical snuffbox
> - tenderness in the scaphoid tubercle
> - pain on compressing the thumb
> - pain on ulnar/radial deviation.

Suspected scaphoid fracture

If a patient presents with the clinical symptoms of a scaphoid fracture but no definite fracture identified on X-ray, it is advisable to treat as a definite scaphoid fracture.

Definite scaphoid fracture

- Scaphoid POP.
- High arm sling for 24 hours.
- Follow-up in fracture clinic.

Old fracture – non-union

Treat as a new scaphoid fracture.

DE QUERVAIN'S TENOSYNOVITIS

This is an inflammatory condition of two specific tendons (abductor pollicis longus and extensor pollicis brevis). It is characterised by a relatively rapid onset of pain around the thumb-side of the wrist which increases in severity on movement of the thumb. A tender swelling is often evident.

This can be an extremely painful condition and the patient will need a lot of reassurance. Treatment is with NSAIDs and a wrist splint. It is important to inform the patient that this may take a few weeks to settle down.

CARPAL TUNNEL SYNDROME

Median nerve dysfunction, median nerve entrapment.

Carpal tunnel syndrome is pressure on the median nerve, which provides feeling and movement to the thumb-side of the hand (the palm, thumb, index finger, middle finger and thumb side of the ring finger). The carpal tunnel, where the nerve enters the hand, is normally narrow, so any swelling can pinch the nerve and cause pain, numbness, tingling or weakness. Patients often complain of severe pain which wakes them up at night.

The condition occurs most often in people 30–60 years old, and is more common in women than men.

It is also associated with other medical problems such as:

- diabetes
- alcoholism
- hypothyroidism
- kidney failure and dialysis
- menopause, premenstrual syndrome and pregnancy
- obesity
- rheumatoid arthritis, systemic lupus erythematosus and scleroderma.

The pain of carpal tunnel syndrome can be reproduced by tapping over the median nerve at the wrist which may cause pain to shoot from the wrist to the hand (this is called Tinel's sign). Also, bending the wrist forward all the way for 60 seconds will usually result in numbness, tingling or weakness (this is called Phalen's test).

UPPER LIMB NEUROPATHIES

Peripheral neuropathy, which is damage to the peripheral nervous system, is not an uncommon presentation; it may be either inherited or acquired. The most likely causes of acquired peripheral neuropathy are:

- trauma
- alcoholism

- diabetes
- vascular disorders.

More complex causes are:
- neoplasms
- autoimmune responses
- nutritional deficiencies.

Radial nerve dysfunction

Damage to the radial nerve leads to problems with movement or sensation of the back of the arm (triceps), forearm or hand. It occurs when there is damage to the radial nerve, which travels down the arm and controls movement of the triceps muscle at the back of the upper arm. This results in diminished sensation in the wrist and hand and an inability to extend the wrist.

Causes include:
- fracture of the humerus
- pressure caused by hanging the arm over the back of a chair (called 'Saturday night palsy' if caused by drinking too much alcohol and falling asleep in that position)
- 'crutch palsy', caused by incorrect use of crutches; this is less common now that elbow crutches are used
- long-term or repeated constriction of the wrist (for example, from wearing a tight watch strap)
- pressure to the upper arm from arm positions during sleep or coma.

Sometimes no cause can be found.

Maintain a high index of suspicion if other nerves are affected as there may be a systemic cause such as diabetes or renal disease.

The following symptoms may occur:
- pain
- abnormal sensations in hand or forearm, dorsal radial aspect of hand
- fingers nearest to the thumb (second and third fingers)
- difficulty extending the arm at the elbow
- difficulty in extending the wrist or even loss of grip
- wrist or finger drop
- paraesthesia, decreased sensation, tingling or burning sensation.

Treatment

In some cases, no treatment is needed and recovery is spontaneous. Over-the-counter analgesics may be adequate but if there is severe neuralgia, anticonvulsant medicines and/or tricyclic antidepressants (amitriptyline) may be needed to reduce nerve pain.

Handcuff neuropathy

The patient may complain of pain around the thumb and residual paraesthesia or decreased sensation over the radial side of the thumb metacarpal due to tight handcuffs.

> ! Patients may ask you to document this injury as evidence of 'police brutality' but it could be due to their own resistance as opposed to too-tight handcuffs. You may be asked to give evidence in court at a later date so make sure your documentation is detailed, accurate and factual (no speculation or personal opinions).

Be careful to examine and document the motor and sensory function of the hand. Draw the area of paraesthesia or decreased sensation.

Reassure the patient and explain that the nerve has been bruised but that its function should return although it may take time.

Consider also other causes such as:

- peripheral neuropathy
- de Quervain's tenosynovitis
- carpal tunnel syndrome
- scaphoid fracture
- gamekeeper's thumb.

Treatment

Simple over-the-counter analgesia may be adequate. Splints may also relieve pain.

CHAPTER 18

Hand injury

The hand is a complex structure where accurate assessment is dependent on sound understanding of the anatomy.

Hand injuries are common in all age groups and call for very careful assessment as subtle injuries to nerves and tendons may not be initially apparent. Misdiagnosis or mismanagement of hand injuries can have serious ramifications for both the patient and the EP's employers.

Be very thorough and methodical in your assessment, documenting positive as well as negative findings. Examine and document nerve, tendon function and vascular status. Always draw diagrams.

Uncomplicated fractures and soft tissue injuries can be initially managed by the EP and followed up in the hand clinic. Complicated injuries should be referred to specialist hand surgeons according to local protocol.

Open fractures, badly contaminated wounds, bite wounds and tendon sheath infections require operative treatment within a few hours and should be referred immediately to hand surgery.

Where there is any doubt, ask for an expert opinion and do not proceed without advice. Document any advice given and from whom.

ASSESSMENT PRIORITIES

- Analgesia.
- Remove rings.
- Elevate in a high sling.

You **must** document:

- mechanism of injury
- time of injury

- dominant hand
- occupation.

Record the presence or absence of tendon activity, nerve function and vascularity.

METACARPAL FRACTURES

Bennett's fracture

Intra-articular fracture/dislocation of the base of the first metacarpal where a small fragment of the first metacarpal continues to articulate with the trapezium. There is also lateral retraction of the first metacarpal shaft by abductor pollicis longus.

Undisplaced Bennett's fracture

- Bennett's POP.
- High arm sling.
- Fracture clinic appointment, next clinic.

Displaced Bennett's fracture

- Analgesia.
- High arm sling.
- Immediate referral to hand surgeons.

Fracture of fifth metacarpal

Fractures of the fifth metacarpal neck are among the most common fractures in the hand. Usually, these fractures are caused by striking a solid object with a closed fist and thus are called boxer's fractures. These fractures are most common in young men.

Check for rotation deformity by asking the patient to flex the fingers to the palm of the hand. All fingers should point towards the thenar eminence and not overlap other fingers.

Refer very displaced fractures, or those where there is significant rotation deformity, to hand surgeons.

Treatment

- Analgesia.
- Volar slab if very swollen or painful, otherwise neighbour strapping.
- High arm sling.
- Fracture clinic appointment, next clinic.

THUMB

Where no bony injury is identified, apply thumb spica and arrange appropriate follow-up.

Hyperextension/hyperabduction injuries

- Pain over base of thumb.
- Loss of grip.
- Instability (no endpoint on stressing).

Rupture of ulnar collateral ligament – skier's thumb, gamekeeper's thumb

This is an injury commonly seen in athletes. Patients typically complain of pain and swelling directly over the torn ligament at the metacarpal phalangeal joint of the thumb. There will be difficulty in grasping objects or holding objects firmly in their grip.

Presence of a Stener lesion suggests complete rupture of the ulnar collateral ligament (UCL). It is characterised by dislocation of the torn end of the ligament dorsally above the adductor aponeurosis/adductor pollicis muscle, such that it is separated from the joint. This impedes healing and is an indication for surgical repair.

Partial tears can be immobilised in a splint and high sling. Complete tears may need surgical intervention. Refer to hand surgeons.

UNDISPLACED FRACTURE – METACARPAL

- Analgesia.
- Bennett's POP.
- If minimal swelling, neighbour strapping.
- High sling and follow-up in fracture clinic.

FRACTURES AND DEFORMITIES OF THE FINGERS

Pain and swelling with no bony injury

- Analgesia.
- High arm sling.
- Early mobilisation.
- Advise patient to see their GP if no improvement within 7–10 days.

Undisplaced fracture – proximal and middle phalanx

- Analgesia.
- Neighbour strapping.

- High arm sling.
- Fracture clinic appointment, next clinic.

Volar plate injury

Hyperextension injury to the proximal interphalangeal joint (PIPJ) causes injury to the volar plate with or without avulsion fracture at the base of the proximal phalanx.

- Neighbour strapping.
- High sling and follow-up with hand surgeons.

Undisplaced fracture – distal phalanx

- Analgesia.
- No splint required.
- Advise patient to avoid contact sports.
- Fracture clinic appointment as appropriate.

Avulsion fracture with extensor tendon injury (mallet deformity)

- Loss of extension at the distal interphalangeal joint (DIPJ) often due to very minor injury.
- Full flexion but loss of extension.
- X-ray to exclude avulsion fracture.
- If no fracture, treat with Zimmer splint and follow up in hand clinic.
- If avulsion fracture present, splint and refer to hand surgeons for ongoing management.
- Advise the patient on the importance of maintaining the finger in extension, particularly if removing the splint to wash the hand.

Displaced fracture – proximal and middle phalanx

Discuss with hand surgeons and treat as advised.

Boutonnière deformity

Rupture or division of the central slip finger extensor tendon following blunt or penetrating trauma.

- Neighbour strapping or boutonnière splint if available.
- High arm sling.
- Refer to hand surgeons.

Swan neck deformity

A swan neck deformity describes a finger with a hyperextended proximal interphalangeal (PIP) joint and a flexed distal interphalangeal (DIP) joint. Chronic inflammation of the PIP joint puts a stretch on the volar plate. Weakness in the volar plate can also occur from a finger injury that forces the PIP joint into hyperextension, stretching or rupturing the volar plate

Trigger finger/thumb (stenosing tenosynovitis)

A painful condition that affects the tendons in the hand. As the finger or thumb is flexed, the tendon gets trapped and the finger clicks or locks.

Around 2–3% of the population develop trigger finger. It is more common in:

- women
- people who are over 40 years of age
- people with certain medical conditions.

In around 20–30% of people, trigger finger may get better without any intervention. For others, surgery is generally the standard treatment.

LACERATIONS AND SOFT TISSUE INJURIES TO THE HAND

Common missed injuries

Nerve injury, pins and needles ignored because of lack of sensory loss.

IMPORTANT

Examine the following structures.

- Median nerve.
- Ulnar nerve.
- Radial nerve.
- Superficial flexor (flexor digitorum superficialis), flexion at PIPJ.
- Deep flexor (flexor digitorum profundus), flexion at DIPJ.
- Extensor tendons.

History

- Time of injury.
- Mechanism of injury.
- Right or left handed.
- Occupation.

Flexor tendon injury

Any significant cut or laceration over the flexor surface of the hand may result in a flexor tendon injury. Examine both flexors carefully and document positive as well as negative findings.

Assess flexor tendons

- Remember to check both flexors to the fingers – two per finger.
- Flexor digitorum profundus – ask patient to flex the finger at the DIPJ to establish integrity of flexor digitorum profundus.
- Flexor digitorum superficialis – assessing this tendon requires more skill as both flexor tendons act on the PIPJ. Asking the patient to flex the PIPJ of the affected finger while holding all other fingers in extension will immobilise all the profundus tendons.

Assess extensor tendons

One per finger with proximal and distal slips. Loss of extensor mechanism will result in a subtle droop of the affected finger.

Digital nerves

- Nerve injuries are not always immediately obvious. It is possible to have significant nerve injuries with minimal or absent signs; there may be only a very slight loss of sensation at the time of first assessment.
- Any reduction or change in sensation of the whole side of the injured finger distal to a cut over a digital nerve suggests damage to the nerve.
- These patients need referral to hand surgeons.

Tendon sheath infection

- Flexor tendon sheath infection is a serious threat to hand function if not identified early and treated.
- Caused by penetrating injury and direct inoculation of bacteria, it usually has a rapid onset.
- Early signs include pain and rapid loss of movement of the affected finger, even before the more typical signs of infection are apparent.
- Infection is in the palmar side of the hand but swelling may be more evident on the dorsal aspect of the hand where the skin is much looser.
- Passive extension of the finger causes particular pain.
- Urgent referral to hand surgeons for surgical drainage is essential.
- Untreated infection may irreparably damage the tendon apparatus, with serious functional consequences.

Amputation of distal phalanx

These injuries can be extremely painful but also very distressing for the patient.

- Ensure adequate analgesia. Opiate analgesia is usually needed.
- X-ray.
- Dress wound loosely in saline-soaked dressing and elevate the arm in a high sling.
- IV antibiotics and tetanus if not fully immunised.
- Place amputated fragment in saline-soaked gauze in a bag of ice.
- Partial or complete amputation needs immediate referral to hand surgery.
- Extensive nail bed damage also needs referral to hand surgeons.

Subungual haematoma

Subungual haematomas are common nail bed injuries caused by blunt or sharp trauma to the fingers or toes. Bleeding from the nail bed results in increased pressure under the nail and can cause significant discomfort.

- Haematoma drainage ('trephining') may relieve pain.
- X-ray the finger to exclude an underlying fracture.
- Fracture is not a contraindication for trephining.
- Check for the presence of an associated extensor tendon injury.
- Haematomas that are larger than 50% of the nail do not necessarily require nail removal and exploration.
- Multiple holes may be necessary to allow adequate drainage.
- Drainage of the subungual haematoma does not expedite healing or prevent infection.
- Trephining is not indicated if the haematoma is not painful.
- Remove acrylic nails if electrocautery is to be used as they may be flammable.

Fingertip injuries

In children, these do remarkably well with minimal treatment. Use Steri-Strips where possible.

Management of superficial injuries

- Anaesthetise with ring block (lidocaine 2% × 5 mL).
- X-ray to exclude fracture.
- Treat with prophylactic antibiotics if fracture present.
- Clean and close lacerations with one or two loose sutures or Steri-Strips.
- Preserve the nail if possible as it acts as a splint.

- Replace the nail if it has flipped out of the base fold and use Steri-Strips to hold in place.
- Establish tetanus status and immunise as needed.
- Finger dressing.
- High sling.
- Elevate and rest.
- Consider review or refer to fracture clinic as appropriate.

CHAPTER 19

Pelvic and femur injuries

COMMON PRESENTATIONS

- Fractured neck of femur.
- Fractured shaft of femur.
- Supracondylar fracture.
- Pubic ramus fracture.
- Ligament sprain.
- Osteoarthritis pain.
- Dislocations.
- Trochanteric bursitis.

IMMEDIATE CHECK

Pelvic and femur fractures are orthopaedic emergencies. Follow ABCs to ensure patient safety and refer for a full medical assessment. Remember the elderly can sustain fractures with relatively minor trauma and may even bear weight on an impacted fractured neck of femur.

- Pain.
- Pallor.
- Pulselessness.
- Paraesthesia.
- Paralysis.

HISTORY

- Describe mechanism of injury.
- Onset/duration of symptoms.
- Site/side.

- Occupation.
- Social history.
- Relevant past medical history.
- Current medications.
- Allergies.

EXAMINATION

Look

- Obvious deformity.
- Bruising.
- Swelling.
- Shortening/external rotation of limb.

Feel

Bony tenderness – iliac crest, greater trochanter, pubic rami, shaft of femur, distal femur, patella, proximal tibia and fibula.

Move

- Abduction and adduction of hip.
- Straight-leg raise.
- Flexion and extension of knee.
- Ability to bear weight.

INVESTIGATIONS

- X-ray hip and pelvis.
- X-ray whole shaft of femur if a fractured shaft of femur is suspected, including knee views.
- Baseline observations.
- FBC, U&E, group and save.

MANAGEMENT

Fractured neck of femur

Most departments will have a fast-track protocol for patients with these injuries.

- IV analgesia.
- Fluids.
- Orthopaedic referral.

Fractured shaft of femur

- IV analgesia.
- Traction such as a Thomas splint or similar can be applied in the ED. This stabilises the fracture, relieves pain and reduces blood loss (recheck distal and proximal pulses, capillary refill and sensation post application).
- Orthopaedic referral.

Supracondylar fracture (distal femur)

- Analgesia.
- Discuss patient with on-call orthopaedic surgeon. Some of these patients are managed conservatively in POP and some require surgery.

Fractured pubic ramus

- Analgesia.
- Attempt mobilisation.
- If possible, these patients can be managed at home with adequate support.
- If not, refer as per local policy for inpatient rehabilitation.
- Always consider the need for extra social support for the elderly patient.

Dislocation of hip

Dislocations of the anatomical hip are rare, and often are a result of major trauma. Dislocations of prosthetic hips more commonly occur.

- Early relocation is required, under sedation in the ED.
- Analgesia.
- X-ray.
- Senior support should be sought to enable reduction.
- Once reduced, the patient will require referral to the on-call orthopaedic team for admission.

Ligament sprain

- Analgesia.
- Mobilisation; consider use of crutches.
- Consider physiotherapy.

Osteoarthritis

- Analgesia.
- Exclude sepsis.
- Mobilisation.
- Advise GP follow-up to obtain orthopaedic outpatient referral.

Trochanteric bursitis

Trochanteric bursitis is a disorder that affects the lateral aspect of the hip or hips. The condition occurs more commonly in women than men and usually affects middle-aged to elderly people.

Causes of the condition include:

- differences in leg length
- a fall on the side of the hip
- repetitive movements
- prolonged or excessive pressure to the hip area
- some infections such as *Staphylococcus* and tuberculosis and diseases like gout and arthritis
- underlying surgical wire, implants or scar tissue in the hip area.

Symptoms

Pain in the thigh and trochanter area. Pain may increase over time and it may last for months. The pain may be more intense when lying on the affected side.

Management

- Rest.
- NSAIDs.
- Physiotherapy.
- Stick (use in hand opposite to affected hip).

CHAPTER 20

Knee injuries

Knee pain may be due to overuse and may be chronic. An overuse injury can also be considered to be acute if it is painful or inflamed.

> IMPORTANT
>
> Musculoskeletal injuries can be very painful and effective analgesia should be ensured prior to examination.

COMMON PRESENTATIONS

- Collateral ligament sprain.
- Twisting injury (menisci).
- Anterior cruciate ligament (ACL) tear.
- Dislocated patella.
- Fractured patella.

Inability to bear weight is suggestive of a significant injury.

COMMONLY MISSED INJURIES

Tibial plateau fracture, neck of fibula fracture (check for foot drop), false-positive bipartite patella.

HISTORY

- Mechanism of injury.
- Time of injury.

- Pain (extreme pain, especially immediately after the injury, may indicate ACL injury).
- An audible pop or crack at the time of injury and a feeling of initial instability may suggest ACL tear.
- Valgus/varus strain.
- Whether swelling was immediate or subsequent (rapid swelling is usually due to haemarthrosis and is suggestive of a significant injury).
- Ask about occupation as limb injuries may adversely affect the patient's ability to look after themselves, i.e. the elderly.
- Past medical history.
- Current medications.
- Known allergies.

EXAMINATION

Look

- Observe gait, limping, partially weight bearing, unable to bear weight.
- Observe and document swelling and bruising.
- Obvious deformity and integrity of skin.
- Restricted movement, especially inability to straighten the leg.
- Patellar effusion.
- Wasting of quadriceps.

To examine the patient properly, he or she must be lying down, with both legs exposed from the hips.

Feel

- Skin temperature, warmth, erythema.
- Popliteal pulses.
- Joint line tenderness.
- Tenderness at the medial side of the joint which may indicate cartilage injury.
- Crepitus.
- Neurovascular deficit.
- Retropatellar crepitus.
- Baker's cyst.

Move

- Medial collateral ligament stress test – laxity/pain.
- Lateral collateral ligament stress test – laxity/pain.

- Straight-leg raise.
- Note any extension block.
- Drawer test.
- McMurray test (meniscus tear). When performed correctly, this is a reliable test for identifying a meniscus tear. However, it is very difficult to perform on a painful swollen knee and probably best left until swelling has subsided.
- Locking.
- Patella apprehension test (obvious apprehension may suggest the patella has recently dislocated).
- Positive signs in the anterior drawer test and Lachman's test may indicate ACL injury.

INVESTIGATIONS

Use the Ottawa Knee Rules to decide whether the patient needs an X-ray. The Ottawa Knee Rules suggest a knee X-ray series is only required for knee injury patients with any of the following findings.

- Age 55 or older.
- Isolated tenderness of the patella (that is, no bone tenderness of the knee other than the patella).
- Tenderness at the head of the fibula.
- Inability to flex to 90°.
- Inability to bear weight both immediately and in the ED (four steps; unable to transfer weight twice onto each lower limb regardless of limping).

MANAGEMENT OF KNEE INJURIES

Acute haemarthrosis

- If tense large swelling (rapid onset) and significant pain, may need aspiration.
- Discuss with ED registrar or orthopaedics.

Bursal swelling

- Prepatellar or infrapatellar, if inflamed.
- Antibiotics, analgesia and review clinic.

Collateral ligament

In the absence of laxity or pain on stressing, ligament injury is unlikely.

Sprained ligament with an effusion

- Rest -Ice - Compression - Elevation.
- Double Tubigrip.
- Crutches.
- Knee injury advice.
- Follow-up in review clinic.

Ligament tear

- Rest -Ice - Compression - Elevation.
- Cricket pad splint.
- Crutches.
- Fracture clinic follow-up.

Femoral condyle fracture

- Refer to orthopaedics.
- Analgesia.
- Elevate.

Patella - undisplaced fracture

- POP cylinder.
- Crutches.
- Fracture clinic appointment.

Patella - displaced fracture

Discuss with orthopaedic registrar and treat as advised.

Patella - dislocation

- If able, reduce the dislocation using Entonox (usually a simple procedure) and apply a POP cylinder/cricket pad splint.
- If not able to reduce, refer to orthopaedic registrar.
- Fracture clinic appointment if reduced, next clinic.

Tibial plateau - undisplaced fracture

- Refer to orthopaedics and treat as advised.
- Application of a long leg above-knee cast, including the foot POP back-slab, is usually advised.

Tibial plateau - displaced fracture

- Refer to orthopaedics.
- Be vigilant for any signs of compartment syndrome.

Tibia – shaft fracture

- Refer to orthopaedics.
- Be vigilant for any signs of compartment syndrome.

Tibia – no bony injury

- Rest –Ice – Compression – Elevation.
- Elastic tubular support.
- Give relevant advice on mobilisation.

Fibula – proximal undisplaced fracture

- Observe any foot drop (unable to hold foot horizontal); suggests peroneal nerve injury.
- Other signs of peroneal nerve injury include:
  - walking abnormalities
  - 'slapping' gait (walking pattern in which each step taken makes a slapping noise)
  - toes drag while walking.
- Check sensation on the dorsal surface of the foot.
- Check for fracture at the ankle joint or swelling over the deltoid ligament which may indicate inferior tibiofibular diastasis.
- Apply a long leg above-knee cast, including the foot POP back-slab.
- Crutches.
- Fracture clinic follow-up.

Fibula – shaft undisplaced fracture

- Check for fracture at the ankle joint or deltoid swelling which suggests disruption of the inferior tibiofibular joint.
- Apply a long leg above-knee cast, including the foot POP back-slab.
- Crutches.
- Fracture clinic follow-up.

Fibula – displaced fracture

- Discuss management with the orthopaedic team.
- Elevate the limb and monitor for signs of compartment syndrome.

Fibula – distal undisplaced fracture

- Below-knee POP back-slab.
- Crutches.
- Fracture clinic follow-up.

CHAPTER 21

Ankle injuries

Ankle injuries are a very common presentation in emergency and urgent care settings. EPs are likely to manage a number of these in any one shift. Familiarity with such injuries can cause complacency, making it easy to miss the subtleties of an individual presentation. Each case should be carefully and objectively assessed.

Ankle dislocation +/– fracture !

This is an orthopaedic emergency and should be reduced immediately with adequate pain relief and, if needed, Entonox, before an X-ray is taken.

Get senior help without delay.

Once reduced, apply a below-knee Plaster of Paris back-slab, then X-ray again. Elevate the limb and check pedal pulses. Definitive management by orthopaedic team.

IMMEDIATE CHECK

- Pain.
- Pallor.
- Pulselessness.
- Paraesthesia.
- Paralysis.

HISTORY

- Describe mechanism of injury.
- Whether able to bear weight immediately after the injury.

- Onset/duration of symptoms (swelling more generalised with delay to presentation).
- Site/side.
- Occupation and hobbies.
- Social history.
- Relevant past medical history.
- Current medications.
- Allergies.

EXAMINATION

Look

- Obvious deformity.
- Colour of skin.
- Erythema.
- Wounds.
- Bruising.
- Swelling.
- Wasting compared to other limb.

Feel

- Skin temperature.
- Pedal pulses.
- Bony tenderness over malleoli, navicular, base of fifth metatarsal and proximal fibula.

Move

- Inversion.
- Eversion.
- Plantarflexion.
- Dorsiflexion.

Ottawa Ankle Rules

Ankle injuries are extremely common but many features on history and physical examination are unreliable. In most cases the decision to X-ray an ankle/foot is made using the Ottawa Ankle Rules.

Although the Rules have a sensitivity of 97.8% and so are a useful tool for determining the need for an X-ray, it is important to remember that every patient is different and rules are not infallible. Therefore act judiciously and use your clinical judgement to decide the best course of action for your patient.

An ankle X-ray is required only if there is any pain in the malleolar zone and any of the following findings:

- bone tenderness at the posterior edge or tip of the lateral malleolus
- bone tenderness at the posterior edge or tip of the medial malleolus
- inability to bear weight both immediately and in the ED.

A foot X-ray is required if there is any pain in the midfoot zone and any of the following findings:

- bone tenderness at the base of the fifth metatarsal
- bone tenderness at the navicular
- inability to bear weight both immediately and in the ED.

MANAGEMENT OF ANKLE INJURIES

Refer any open or displaced fractures or neurovascular damage immediately to the ED senior doctor or orthopaedics. Avoid delays as fracture blisters can develop very quickly.

Bimalleolar/trimalleolar fractures

- Analgesia.
- Splint.
- Refer to orthopaedics.

Undisplaced fracture of distal tibia

- Analgesia.
- Check stability of ankle joint. Discuss with orthopaedics.
- Above-knee Plaster of Paris.
- Crutches (patient to be non-weight bearing).
- Appointment at next fracture clinic.

Undisplaced distal fibular fracture

- Analgesia.
- Below-knee back-slab.
- Crutches (patient to be non-weight bearing).
- Appointment at next fracture clinic.

Avulsion fracture of distal fibula

- Depending on the degree of pain and swelling, this can be treated as a severe sprain.

- Elastic bandage, non-weight bearing and crutches.
- Follow-up in fracture clinic.

Achilles tendon injuries

- Common injury in middle-aged males.
- Assess extent of injury:
  - feel for a palpable gap along the tendon
  - Simmond's test (loss of plantarflexion on squeezing calf).
- **Note:** may still be able to stand on tip toes if tibialis posterior and peroneal and toe flexor muscles are still intact.

Treatment of ruptured tendon

Immediate review by orthopaedics is indicated if torn. Some centres may admit the patient for surgical repair.

Management of partial tears should include:

- analgesia
- equinus POP
- crutches
- plaster advice and instructions
- follow-up in fracture clinic.

MANAGEMENT OF SPRAINED LIGAMENTS

Treatment for ligament injuries should include splinting and RICER (rest, ice, compression, elevation and rehabilitation). Exclude a complete tear of the calcaneo-fibular and talo-fibular ligaments by peforming a drawer testing of the ankle before discharging the patient.

Treatment will depend on the grade of the sprain.

Grade 1 – simple sprains

- Aim – reduce swelling and pain.
- Analgesia.
- Early mobilisation.
- Rest (with foot elevated for 24–48 hours).
- Ice.
- Compression.
- Elevation.
- Rehabilitation (encourage normal mobilisation after 48 hours).

Grade 2 – moderate sprains

- As for grade 1 sprain.
- Analgesia.

- If patient unable to bear weight, crutches may be required.
- Physiotherapy referral should be immediate or not at all.
- Review in one week if symptoms do not resolve.

Grade 3 – severe sprains

- Depending on clinical examination, these patients may need an X-ray.
- Pain relief.
- Support.
- Rehabilitation.
- Refer to physiotherapy.
- Give advice on ice/massage/elevation.
- Crutches will be needed.

CHAPTER 22

Foot injuries

Injuries to the feet are often associated with ankle injury but can also be isolated.

Easily missed or misdiagnosed fractures are Lisfranc and Jones fractures.

HISTORY

- Mechanism of injury.
- Associated with ankle injury.
- Fall from height (consider calcaneum and associated spinal injury).
- Ability to bear weight since injury.
- Consider stress fractures.
- Occupation.
- Past medical history.
- Medications.
- Allergies.

TARSAL BONES – ALL FRACTURES

- Non-weight bearing.
- Below-knee POP back-slab.
- Crutches.
- Fracture clinic next appointment.

If suspicious of calcaneum fracture, request calcaneal views.

CALCANEUM FRACTURES

Consider injury to lumbar spine.

- Discuss management with the orthopaedic registrar.
- Treat as advised.

METATARSALS

Undisplaced fractures

- Below-knee POP back-slab.
- Crutches.
- Fracture clinic appointment, next clinic.

Avulsion fracture of the base of the fifth metatarsal

- Below-knee POP back-slab if severe swelling and discomfort, otherwise
- Elastic support bandage.
- Crutches.
- Fracture clinic follow-up.

LISFRANC FRACTURE

Lisfranc joint injuries are rare, complex and often misdiagnosed or inadequately treated. Lisfranc injuries can vary from simple ligament tears to complete disruption of the tarsometatarsal (TMT) joint. These injuries are often mistaken for sprains as they are often difficult to see on X-rays. Unrecognised Lisfranc injuries can have serious complications such as joint degeneration and compartment syndrome, which can damage nerve cells and blood vessels. Maintain a high index of suspicion if pain is disproportionate to the clinical picture.

Displaced fracture of metatarsal

- When more than one metatarsal is fractured, check the alignment.
- Discuss with the orthopaedic team.
- Treat as advised.

JONES FRACTURE

Jones fractures occur in a small area of the fifth metatarsal that receives less blood and is therefore more difficult to heal. A Jones fracture can be either a stress fracture or an acute (sudden) break. Jones fractures are caused by overuse, repetitive stress or trauma. They are less common and more difficult to treat than avulsion fractures.

PLANTAR FASCIITIS

Plantar fasciitis is a common, painful foot condition. Plantar fasciitis refers to the syndrome of inflammation of the band of tissue that runs from the heel along the arch of the foot. About 70% of patients with plantar fasciitis have been noted to have a heel spur that can be seen on X-ray of the lateral aspect of the calcaneum.

Treatment

- Rest.
- Non-steroidal anti-inflammatory analgesia.
- Heel support.
- Advice leaflet.

MORTON'S NEUROMA

Morton's neuroma is an intermetatarsal neuroma which occurs between the third and fourth toes. Symptoms, which may begin gradually, may include:

- pain
- a sensation of a foreign body in the ball of the foot
- burning, or numbness and tingling.

Treatment initially is conservative, including rest and NSAID medication. If the pain does not resolve and becomes incapacitating to the patient, surgical excision may be indicated.

CHAPTER 23

Toe injuries

COMMON PRESENTATIONS

- ➤ Fractures.
- ➤ Wounds.
- ➤ Nail bed injuries.

Very careful consideration needs to be given to the management of diabetic foot injuries.

IMMEDIATE CHECK

- ➤ Pain.
- ➤ Pallor.
- ➤ Pulselessness.
- ➤ Paraesthesia.
- ➤ Paralysis.

HISTORY

- ➤ Describe mechanism of injury.
- ➤ Onset/duration of symptoms.
- ➤ Site/side.
- ➤ Occupation.
- ➤ Social history.
- ➤ Relevant past medical history (especially diabetes/peripheral vascular disease).
- ➤ Current medications.
- ➤ Allergies.

EXAMINATION

Look

- Deformity.
- Wounds.
- Bruising.
- Swelling.

Feel

- Skin temperature.
- Sensation.
- Bony tenderness.

INVESTIGATIONS

X-ray, generally only if great toe or suspected dislocation/displaced fracture. Follow local guidelines.

MANAGEMENT

Fracture of small toes (non-displaced or suspected fracture)

- Analgesia.
- Neighbour strap if necessary.
- Advise patient to wear comfortable shoes.
- Generally no further follow-up required.

Dislocation/displacement

- Analgesia.
- Neurovascular assessment.
- Local anaesthetic (nerve block) +/– Entonox.
- Relocate/realign.
- Immobilise/splint.
- X-ray again.
- Recheck neurovascular status.
- Follow up as per local policy.

Great toe

- As above, but usually with fracture clinic follow-up.
- Consider toe spica with Elastoplast.
- Consider need for crutches.

Wounds

- Careful consideration should be given to the mechanism of injury and the indication for prophylactic antibiotics.
- Check neurovascular status.
- X-ray wounds if radio-opaque foreign body suspected.
- Tetanus status should be assessed and prophylaxis given as needed.
- Good wound toileting and appropriate closure/dressing utilised.
- The use of crutches should be considered, particularly if the wound is on the plantar aspect of the foot.

CHAPTER 24

Paediatric fractures and dislocations

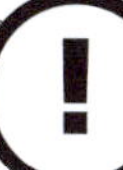

Always ensure analgesia and use distraction when examining small children.

- Fractures are painful and can be the cause of great distress to both child and parents so give adequate analgesia.
- Immobilise as soon as possible.
- Always check and document neurovascular status.
- Be mindful of NAI, especially if the child is <2 years.

Greenstick fracture, also known as a buckle fracture or torus fracture, is a fracture of children. The bone is broken but the periosteum remains intact. It is a common fracture of the forearm in early childhood, usually the result of a fall onto an outstretched hand. These fractures are often missed due to the subtlety of presentation. Signs include:

- tenderness over the distal radius
- reluctance to use the affected limb
- minimal swelling.

X-ray full arm and clavicle to exclude associated fracture.

TODDLER FRACTURE

Non-displaced oblique fracture of the distal tibia in children, nine months to three years of age. May present with an acute onset of limp or refusal to bear weight on one leg. Parents are often unsure of what happened, which may raise suspicion of NAI. Emergency nurse practitioners need to be careful when considering the possibility of NAI, weighing up this possibility against the various conditions that can be mistaken for abuse.

Signs of a toddler's fracture can be subtle, with non-specific physical findings of local injury. Radiological signs can also be subtle.

Management

- Analgesia.
- POP cylinder.
- Fracture clinic appointment.

GROWTH PLATE INJURIES

These injuries are peculiar to children. They were classified into five types by Salter and Harris (1963).

SUPRACONDYLAR FRACTURE OF THE HUMERUS

A supracondylar fracture is a fracture of the distal humerus just above the elbow joint. It is caused by a fall on the outstretched hand with a hyperextension force acting on the elbow.

- Common fracture in children aged 5–9 years.
- Twice as common in boys.

Symptoms include:

- pain
- swelling
- deformity at the elbow region.

In undisplaced fractures, swelling and pain may be minimal with tenderness only over the fracture site. Due to the presence of mild symptoms, diagnosis may be delayed as the parents may not suspect a fracture and report late.

In displaced fractures the deformity is obvious.

> **!** Important nerves and blood vessels present near the elbow joint may be injured by a displaced fracture. The brachial artery may be trapped so regular radial pulse check is imperative until definite management is instituted.

Management

- Analgesia.
- Splint/broad arm sling.
- Refer to orthopaedics.

PULLED ELBOW IN A CHILD

- Presents with a history of not using the arm.
- Examination shows no obvious deformity but a limp arm with pain on supination.
- Reduce by supination while axial compression is applied to forearm. Usually a click is felt.
- Try to distract the child while reducing the elbow.
- If unable to reduce, request orthopaedic review.

Reference

Salter RB, Harris WR. Injuries involving the epiphyseal plate. *J Bone Joint Surg*. 1963; **45A**: 587–622.

CHAPTER 25

Limping child

A limping child is a common presentation in emergency/urgent care settings. Some will have a preceding history of injury, but often this is not the case so careful history taking and thorough examination are essential so as not to miss serious pathology.

A knowledge of the possible differential diagnoses is essential in guiding accurate history taking and examination. These presentations can be complicated so maintain a high index of suspicion and low threshold for referral for specialist opinion. In case of doubt, always ask for help.

IMPORTANT CONSIDERATIONS FOR NON-ACCIDENTAL INJURY

- History not consistent with injury or age of child.
- Delay in attendance.
- Repeat attendance due to trauma/different injuries.
- Not living locally, no explanation for attendance.
- Strained relationship between child and parent/carer.
- Inappropriate behaviour.

HISTORY

- Indicate source.
- History of trauma.
- Duration of problem.
- Type of pain (worse at night/morning, provocation/palliation).
- Past medical history.
- Family history.
- Social history.
- Medication (what medications have been taken to relieve the pain).
- Allergies.

EXAMINATION

Look

- Vital signs.
- With child standing, check for scoliosis.
- Pelvic tilt.
- Gait (walking on heels, walking on toes).

Feel

- Measure and compare leg lengths.
- Look for asymmetry.
- Check pulses in both legs (femoral, popliteal, anterior tibial, posterior tibial, dorsalis).
- Check patellar and ankle reflexes.

Move

	Right	*Normal range (degrees)*	*Left*
Hip			
Flexion		0–120	
Extension		0–30	
Abduction		0–40	
Adduction		0–30	
Internal rotation		0–40	
External rotation		0–40	
Knee			
Flexion		0–120	
Extension		0 (full extension is 0°)	
Ankle			
Dorsiflexion		0–20	
Plantarflexion		0–50	
Inversion		0–20	
Eversion		0–15	
Pulses			
Femoral			
Popliteal			
Anterior tibial			
Posterior tibial			
Dorsalis pedis			
Reflexes			
Patellar			
Ankle			

INVESTIGATIONS

- FBC/ESR/CRP/blood culture if pyrexial and infection likely.
- Sickle cell screen if appropriate.
- X-rays. Screening views including pelvis and whole limb in small children.

MANAGEMENT

- Analgesia.
- Refer any suspected cases of NAI to paediatrics immediately.

Conditions requiring urgent paediatric assessment

- Septic arthritis.
- Slipped upper femoral epiphysis (SUFE).
- Dislocation of hip.
- Sickle cell crisis.

Serious pathology to consider if no history of trauma and sudden onset

Septic arthritis

- Any age.
- Generally unwell/pyrexia. Temperature >38°.
- Signs of inflammation.
- Severe pain on passive internal rotation of hips.

Transient synovitis of hip (irritable hip)

- From 18 months to 12 years old.
- Normal FBC, ESR, CRP and apyrexial, history >2 weeks preceded by viral infection.
- Pain on passive internal rotation.

Perthes' disease

- From two to 10 years old.
- Male, thin, shorter than average.
- Pain in hip or referred to thigh or knee.
- Limited and painful internal rotation.
- Shortened leg.

Slipped upper femoral epiphysis

- From 10 to 18 years old.
- Male, overweight.
- May give a history of trauma.

- Painful hip.
- Some complain of knee pain.
- Limited and painful internal rotation and flexion.
- Shortened leg.

Sickle cell disease

- Six months to five years old.
- Antalgic gait.
- Refusing to bear weight.
- Raised inflammatory markers.

Non-acute onset

Juvenile rheumatoid arthritis

- From two to 10 years old.
- Generally symmetrical but could begin as a monoarthritis.
- Fever and raised inflammatory markers.

Osgood–Schlatter disease

- 10–16 years old.
- History of trauma or sport related.
- Prominent and painful tibial tuberosity.

Congenital dislocation of hip

- Birth to two years.
- Shorter leg.
- Skinfold discrepancy (skinfolds in the thighs will appear uneven).
- Reduction in external rotation and abduction.

Length discrepancy

- No pain.
- No clinical findings.

Other causes

- 'Growing pains'.
- Myopathies.
- Muscular dystrophy.
- Guillain–Barré syndrome.
- Rickets.
- Appendicitis.
- Psychomatic.

MANAGEMENT

- All these conditions will require specialist paediatric referral.
- The role of the EP is to reassure and advise parents and carers.
- Ensure analgesia.
- Refer to paediatric specialist for further investigation and management.

SECTION 3
Skin

CHAPTER 26

Skin trauma

COMMON PRESENTATIONS

- Lacerations to head, face and limbs.
- Animal/human bites.
- Burns/scalds.
- Foreign bodies.

IMMEDIATE CHECK

- Arrest haemorrhage. Apply pressure.
- Assess and document GCS in any scalp laceration.
- Check the 5Ps in any limb laceration: pain, pallor, pulse, paraesthesia, paralysis.
- Consider deep structural injury in any skin trauma.
- Remember that puncture wounds in the proximal forearm can damage the brachial artery and lead to compartment syndrome.
- Note any history of spurting blood loss and/or severe pain.

COMMON PROBLEMS ASSOCIATED WITH SKIN TRAUMA

- Infection due to poor debridement, particularly if effective local anaesthesia is not achieved.
- Nerve injury, report of paraesthesia not heeded because of lack of objective loss of sensation.
- Tendon injury: flexor digitorum superficialis injury.
- Consider joint penetration where laceration lies over a joint.
- Keloid scarring in darker skins.

HISTORY

- Indicate source of history if not patient.
- Age, occupation.
- Date and time of injury.
- Mechanism.
- Site.
- Dominant hand.
- Last meal.
- Past medical history (relevant illnesses, diabetes).
- Allergies.
- Medication.

EXAMINATION

- All findings must be documented and illustrated where possible.
- Define complexity of laceration.
- Exclude underlying injury.
- Haemorrhage.
- Skin loss.
- Dirty wound.
- Irregular skin edge.
- Deep fascia breached.
- Assume that glass has cut through skin and bone.
- Loss of sensation.
- Weakness/numbness/paraesthesia may indicate nerve injury/vascular injury.
- Vascular injury (capillary fill, distal pulse, colour).
- Check flexor/extensors in finger/hand lacerations.
- Foreign bodies (FB)/glass (indicate site, size, number of FB).
- Puncture wound may need exploration.
- Consider bony involvement.

INVESTIGATIONS

- Always X-ray for glass, metal or tooth fragments (or other radio-opaque FB).
- In some circumstances, a check X-ray may be indicated following removal of the FB.
- If glass FB is tiny and unable to be removed, leave *in situ* and suture laceration.
- If wounds are bleeding profusely, apply pressure and elevate, consider the need for FBC, group and save and fluid replacement.

SUTURING

This handbook assumes proficiency in suturing/wound closure so the following points are intended as an *aide-mémoire*.

Analgesia in wound management

- Ensure that the patient has had adequate analgesia before attempting to clean the wound as it is difficult to clean a wound thoroughly if the patient is wincing and in pain.
- For deeper wounds, infiltrate with local anaesthetic.
- Anaesthetise with 1% plain lidocaine (maximum dose 3 mg/kg).
- Use digital block if laceration to finger/thumb. Use 2% lidocaine up to 5 mL.
- Document amount of lidocaine used.
- Clean thoroughly and debride, if necessary.
- Ensure effective analgesia before attempting to suture.
- Select appropriate suture material.
- Document number of sutures used.

Suture material

- Scalp – 3/0; removal of suture 7 days.
- Face – 5/0; removal of suture 3–5 days.
- Hands – 4/0; removal of suture 10 days.
- Trunk/limbs – 3/0 or 4/0; removal of suture 10 days.

IMPORTANT

- Never suture tightly.
- If the wound is wide and gaping, consider the need for subcutaneous sutures.
- Aim for opposition of skin edges and always be alert for potential swelling, especially in digits.
- **Never use adrenaline with lidocaine for extremities.**

Cautions

As a general rule, wounds that should not be sutured are:

- animal/human bites (clean thoroughly + antibiotics: co-amoxiclav, erythromycin or metronidazole)
- pretibial lacerations in the elderly (Steri-Strip)
- very dirty wounds
- wounds more than 12 hours old (consider delayed secondary suture, except face).

Aftercare

- Prescribe and administer tetanus prophylaxis, if required.
- Apply non-adhesive dressing.
- Always apply a high arm sling for upper limb injuries.
- Educate patient regarding wound management, provide wound care leaflet.
- Give advice re scarring and risk of infection: any wound can scar and scarring is unpredictable.
- Risk of scarring increased if Afro-Caribbean (keloid formation), skin/crush injury, contaminated wound, irregular skin edges, previous scarring.
- Letter to general practitioner/practice nurse for removal of suture(s).

MANAGEMENT

Specific lacerations

- **Tendon/nerve/vascular.** Refer to plastics/vascular as appropriate.
- **Complex facial laceration.** Refer to maxillofacial surgeons.
- **Eyelid/tarsal plate involvement.** Refer to ophthalmologists.
- **Lacerations to the tongue** need suturing if the wound is wide and gaping and should be sutured by a clinician competent to do so.
- **Lacerations through the vermilion border** of the lip need suturing.
- **Wounds to the face** should be sutured using 5/0 non-absorbable nylon suture. Minimise scarring by thorough wound toilet, including debridement of damaged or necrotic tissue. Consider the need for prophylactic antibiotics in contaminated wounds.

Foreign body in wounds

- Where possible, remove foreign bodies from an open wound if easy or if competent to do so.
- Consider the likelihood of deep injury and infection if FB is associated with a laceration.
- Every attempt should be made to remove FBs.

Foreign body with no open wound

- Refer to ED review clinic or orthopaedics.
- Consider antibiotics if any evidence of infection.

Removal of fish hook from finger

- If pain severe and hook embedded, use digital nerve block.
- Gently push hook forward and out through skin.

- Antibiotics are rarely needed.
- Ensure tetanus immunisation.

Removal of earring or earring back from earlobe

It is not unusual for either an earring or the earring back to become embedded in the earlobe.

This is more likely to occur soon after first piercing of the earlobe and in younger patients. If the ear lobe is very swollen and painful then it will be necessary to use local anaesthetic and make a small incision over the posterior aspect of the earlobe to remove the FB.

Injuries from glass

- May present with severe pain.
- Ensure the patient is given analgesia prior to examination.
- Remember that puncture wounds in limbs may damage arteries and lead to compartment syndrome.
- Give due consideration to a history of spurting blood loss.
- Paraesthesia, skin mottling or pain extending to fingers are all signs suggestive of neurovascular injury – be cautious of diagnosis and refer to plastics/hand surgery.
- Assume that glass has cut through skin, nerves and tendons and injured bone. Examine carefully.
- X-ray for glass FB.
- If glass FB is tiny and unable to be removed, leave *in situ* and suture laceration.
- Inform patient that the FB is still in place.

Pretibial lacerations

Pretibial lacerations are a common presentation, particularly in elderly women.

- Sometimes associated with long-term corticosteroid treatment.
- Healing may be impaired and very slow.
- Skilled initial management can have successful outcomes.
- On first examination, the wound flap often appears concertina-ed backwards, leaving a deep open wound.
- The flap needs to be gently smoothed over the wound after gentle cleansing with saline and removal of any haematoma.
- The skin edges of the flap should be brought together and Steri-Stripped.
- These wounds should not be sutured; this can lead to necrosis of the flap.
- Cover the wound with a non-adherent, well-padded dressing and a support bandage. Apply toe-to-knee bandage to encourage even circulation.

- Advise the patient to mobilise as necessary but also to elevate the limb where possible to aid venous return and to prevent the development of a chronic, non-healing leg ulcer.
- Consider tetanus status and the need for antibiotic prophylaxis.
- Simple analgesia such as paracetamol is advisable to control any pain.
- Discharge into the care of the GP and practice nurse is the most appropriate option, where continuity of care is more likely than in hospital.
- Consider early referral to plastic surgeons for skin grafting for patients with skin loss to optimise outcomes.
- Health promotion in this group of patients is paramount to prevent chronic non-healing.
- Assessment of the patient holistically and not the wound in isolation is the gold standard and will promote successful treatment.
- Consider referral to occupational therapy in line with local policy to provide added support.
- Also consider referral to falls clinic.

CHAPTER 27

Burns and scalds

GET SENIOR HELP IMMEDIATELY FOR THE FOLLOWING

- Airway complications.
- Inhalation burns/respiratory distress.
- Burns covering more than 10% body surface area (BSA) in an adult and >5% in a child.
- Full-thickness burns.
- Primary area burn (face, palm, sole, genitals).
- Circumferential burns.
- Electrical burns.
- NAI.

PRINCIPLES OF FIRST AID

- Stop the burning process and cool the wound.
- The burn surface should be cooled with cold running water.
- Analgesia should also be given as soon as possible.

HISTORY

- The history of the incident is essential. How did the burn occur and with what? The cause of the burn will give some indication as to whether the burn is likely to be superficial or deep.
- Scald burns are usually superficial whilst flame burns are likely to be deep, especially if flammable solvents were involved.
- If the patient is a child or elderly consider NAI and elder abuse.
- Time of incident.
- Immediate action/first aid measures taken.
- Past medical history.
- Medication history, especially tetanus status.
- Known allergies.

EXAMINATION

Carefully assess the burn using the Rule of Nines and document the appearance. The palmar surface of the hand (from fingertips to wrist is approximately 1% of BSA) can also be used as a guide to assess small or patchy burns.

Wherever possible, draw diagrams and record:

- colour of burn
- presence or absence of blistering
- presence or absence of sensation to fine pinprick
- presence or absence of capillary refill following digital pressure
- level of pain
- nature of any exudates (may suggest infection in a delayed presentation)
- presence or absence of surrounding inflammation.

Table 27.1 Diagnosis of burn depth

Depth	*Colour*	*Blisters*	*Capillary refill*	*Sensation*	*Healing*
Epidermal 1st degree, e.g. sunburn	Red	No	Present	Present	Yes
Superficial dermal 2nd degree	Pale pink	Yes/small	Present	Present	Yes
Deep dermal 2nd degree	Blotchy red	+/–	Variable	Variable	Very variable
Full thickness 3rd degree	White	No	Absent	Absent	No

CHEMICAL BURNS

Tissue damage as a result of chemical exposure will be difficult to estimate in the first few hours and will be dependent on:

- strength and quantity of the agent
- manner and duration of skin contact
- extent of penetration into tissue
- mechanism of action.

The main difference between chemical and thermal burns is the length of time tissue destruction continues as the chemical agent causes progressive damage until it is inactivated either by a neutralising agent or dilution with water. Alkalis are worse than acid.

First aid

- Constant irrigation with cold running water is the treatment for most chemical burns (except elemental sodium, potassium and lithium).

- Try to establish what the agent was and consult TOXBASE or the National Poisons Information Service for further information.
- Discuss management with the local burns unit.

MANAGEMENT OF MINOR BURNS

- Gently clean the wound with saline. Aseptic technique is essential to minimise the risk of further contamination and care should be taken to avoid further tissue damage.
- Small blisters may be left intact but burst blisters and concertina-ed dead skin should be gently removed.
- Apply occlusive dressings in accordance with local protocol or as advised by burns unit.
- Burns which appear infected at initial presentation or have been contaminated should be dressed with an antimicrobial agent. Such dressings need to be changed daily.
- Burns of the hand: dress with liquid paraffin and cover with a plastic glove or bag.
- Facial burns: clean with normal saline and leave exposed.
- Vaseline for lips.
- Sterile liquid paraffin for creases only.
- Reassure and advise the patient of the likely course and duration of the healing period and that the burn may appear worse before it begins to heal.
- Check tetanus status and immunise as required.
- Ensure the patient is discharged with adequate analgesia.

REFERRAL CRITERIA

Most minor burns can be managed locally. The British Burn Association has identified the following as those that require referral to a burns unit.

- Burns greater than 10% total BSA.
- Burns of special areas: face, hands, feet, genitalia, perineum and major joints.
- Full-thickness burns greater than 5% total BSA.
- Electrical burns.
- Chemical burns.
- Burns with associated inhalational injury.
- Circumferential burns to limbs or chest.
- Burns at the extremes of age.
- Burns in patients with pre-existing medical conditions which could complicate management.
- Any burn patient with associated trauma.

CHAPTER 28

Animal and human bites

Severe infection/cellulitis as a result of a bite may need admission for IV antibiotics.

Human bite injuries may result in litigation so make sure your notes are detailed and comprehensive as you may be called to give evidence in court at a later date. Draw diagrams wherever you can.

HISTORY

- Bite injury – animal/insect/human.
- Time of injury.
- Any associated injury.
- Onset of symptoms.
- Tetanus status.
- Past medical history.
- Allergies.

EXAMINATION

- Signs of systemic allergic reaction, i.e. mucosal swelling, difficulty in breathing, signs of shock.
- Pyrexia.
- Area of erythema, swelling, tenderness.
- Obvious infection/tracking.
- If a human bite, consider the likelihood of a retained tooth and X-ray to exclude FB.

MANAGEMENT

Human bite

- Clean wound thoroughly and apply antibacterial type dressing.
- Tetanus prophylaxis.
- Antibiotics (follow local guidelines, including anaerobes).
- Consider the need for hepatitis B prophylaxis.
- Evaluate the risk of HIV. Refer to the local needlestick/sharps injury policy or discuss management with specialist as appropriate.
- Bites to the face may need referral to maxillofacial/plastic surgeons to ensure optimum cosmetic outcomes.

Animal bite

- Clean thoroughly.
- Ensure no FB in wound.
- Antibacterial dressing.
- Tetanus prophylaxis.
- Antibiotics (including anaerobes).
- Discuss options for closure with senior clinician with due consideration to cosmetic outcome.

Insect bites

- Clean wound thoroughly.
- Antibacterial dressing.
- Tetanus prophylaxis.
- Antihistamine.
- Antibiotics if infected.
- If there is a recent history of foreign travel and the patient is pyrexial and unwell, consider infectious disease.
- Refer for medical assessment.

Management of superficial bites

- Clean thoroughly.
- Dressing (antibacterial).
- Elevate/rest according to affected area.
- Check tetanus status and consider tetanus immunoglobulin in accordance with tetanus protocol.
- Hepatitis B prophylaxis if needed.
- Antibiotic prophylaxis.
- Educate patient regarding signs and symptoms of further infection and emphasise the importance of review of the wound.
- Most bites should be reviewed the following day.
- Consider referral to a doctor if there are signs of cellulitis or lymphangitis.

Removal of ticks

The main aim is to remove all parts of the tick to prevent it releasing additional saliva or regurgitating its stomach contents into the bite wound.

- With a splinter forceps or pointed tweezers, grasp the tick as close to the skin as possible without squeezing the tick's body.
- Pull the tick out without twisting; this may be difficult.
- If you do not have a tweezers use a cotton thread.
- Tie a single loop of cotton around the tick's mouthparts, as close to the skin as possible, then pull gently upwards and outwards.
- Do not squeeze or twist the body of the tick, as this may cause the head and body to separate, leaving the head embedded in the skin.
- After tick removal, cleanse the bite site and dispose of the tweezers. Wash hands thoroughly afterwards.
- Check tetanus status.

Bed bugs

Bed bugs, which are increasingly common, are most active at night and bite any exposed areas of skin while an individual is asleep. The face, neck, hands and arms are common sites for bed bug bites.

- Small, flat or raised bumps on the skin are the most common sign; redness, swelling and itching also occur.
- No treatment is required for bed bug bites. If itching is severe, steroid creams or oral antihistamines may be used for symptom relief.
- Fumigation of the room may be required to eradicate the infestation.

CHAPTER 29

Skin infections

Skin infections of varying degrees of severity are a common presentation in emergency and urgent care settings.

Consider referral to the medical team of any patient with a skin infection who:

- is systemically unwell
- is already on oral antibiotics and not improving
- has diabetes
- is immunosuppressed/neutropenic.

Patients who are pyrexial and systemically unwell with skin infections may need admission for IV antibiotics.

COMMON PRESENTATIONS

- Cellulitis.
- Impetigo.
- Abscesses, which include:
  - **furuncles** – inflammation of a hair follicle
  - **carbuncle** – a cluster of interconnected boils.
- Infected sebaceous cysts.
- Paronychia.

HISTORY

- Onset and duration of presenting complaint.
- Any history of trauma, wound or source of infection, FB.
- Any long-standing skin condition, i.e. eczema.
- Pain and nature of pain.
- Throbbing pain, lack of sleep.

- Past medical history; consider diabetes.
- Drug history (bear in mind skin reactions due to drugs).
- Known allergies.

EXAMINATION

- Patient appearance – flushed, distressed, obvious rash or skin infection.
- Site and extent of erythema.
- Warmth and swelling at site.
- Tracking of erythema (lymphangitis).
- Localised collection, induration, pointing, fluctuant, pus noted.
- Swelling and tenderness over a joint.
- Systemic symptoms, tachycardia.

INVESTIGATIONS

- X-ray if any suspicion of FB.
- Capillary blood glucose estimation for all skin infections.
- FBC, U&E, CRP and blood cultures if patient is systemically unwell.
- Swab any exudates for culture and sensitivity.
- Demarcate area with indelible ink.

ABSCESS

- All abscesses should be drained the same day.
- Refer genital, breast, perianal, pilonidal, facial, neck and labial abscesses to surgeons/gynaecologists.
- If unsure/site difficult, ask for senior help.
- Consider also infected sebaceous cyst, sinus, systemic infection, cellulitis, FB, skin lumps.

Management of abscesses

Always check for diabetes mellitus (capillary blood glucose).

Incision and drainage

- Ensure adequate anaesthesia, injected circumferentially around the abscess.
- This can be a very painful procedure so use Entonox breathed for two minutes prior to the incision. This will relieve pain and also divert the patient's focus from the abscess.
- Make an incision which will allow drainage.
- Express all the pus and curette gently.
- Irrigate the cavity with saline and pack with a hydrophilic dressing.

Aftercare

Re-dress the next day and refer the patient back to the GP.

INFECTED SEBACEOUS CYSTS

Treat as for abscesses.

CELLULITIS

- Exclude diabetes mellitus.
- Look for and document site of entry.
- Mark edge of erythema with a pen so that resolution can be monitored.
- Elevation of limb, higher than the heart.
- Advise patient to rest affected part.
- If severe or patient systemically unwell with temperature >38°, consider referral/admission.
- Consider the need for tetanus immunisation.
- Treat with antibiotics according to local guidelines.
- Arrange to review the patient the following day or advise them to visit their GP if symptoms are not resolving or become more severe.

PARONYCHIA

- If pus is localised and obvious, incise to express all the pus.
- Remove overlying skin if lifted off.
- If pus is present on the nail bed, remove part of the nail to allow drainage. Sometimes trephining will suffice.
- Review according to severity or refer back to GP.

PULP INFECTIONS

THESE PATIENTS NEED URGENT REFERRAL TO A HAND SURGEON

The pulp of a finger is divided into many small fatty compartments by strands of fibrous tissue which run from the skin to the periosteum of the terminal phalanx. There is little room for swelling, so any infection in the pulp aspect will give rise to early throbbing pain. Pus from the pulp can track through the periosteum, causing osteomyelitis of the distal phalanx. These patients need urgent referral to hand surgery.

IMPETIGO

- Impetigo is a contagious bacterial infection of the surface layers of the skin caused by either *Streptococcus* or *Staphylococcus*.
- Most commonly, it affects children because of their daily environments, such as schools and nurseries, where infection can spread easily, but it sometimes affects adults, especially where people are living together in crowded living conditions.
- Impetigo is divided into two categories:
  - non-bullous impetigo is the most common type which causes sores that quickly rupture, leaving a yellow-brown crust
  - bullous impetigo, which causes large, painless, fluid-filled blisters.
- Treatment is usually with penicillin and antibiotic creams are also recommended. The patient and carers must be advised to wash hands after touching affected areas of skin, and not share towels or bed linen to avoid spreading the infection. Patients should be reassured that impetigo is a self-limiting condition and only very rarely does it spread to cause a cellulitis.

SCABIES

- Scabies is a contagious skin condition whose main symptom is relentless itching. It is caused by tiny mites called *Sarcoptes scabiei,* which burrow into the skin.
- Scabies can be spread through:
  - skin-to-skin contact for long periods of time with someone who is infected
  - sexual contact with someone who is infected.
- Scabies can also be passed on through sharing clothing, towels and bedding with someone who is infected.
- Scabies like warm places on the skin, such as skinfolds, between the fingers, under fingernails or around the buttock or breast creases. They can also be found under watch straps.
- Treatment is with permethrin 5% dermal cream; for those allergic to permethrin, a lotion called malathion 0.5% aqueous liquid can be used. Both of these products can be bought over the counter in pharmacies.

SECTION 4

Ophthalmology

CHAPTER 30

Eyes

Eye problems are a common presentation in the emergency and urgent care settings. As access to specialist ophthalmology is not always immediate, it is essential that ENPs, particularly those working in stand-alone or nurse-led units, are competent to safely assess and differentiate between the acute and urgent cases and those that can be seen more routinely.

COMMON PRESENTATIONS

Injuries

- Chemical injuries.
- Corneal abrasions.
- Subtarsal FB.
- Corneal FB.
- Hyphaema.
- Black eye.
- Eyelid lacerations.
- Open eye trauma.
- Orbital trauma.
- Retinal detachment.

Infections

- Conjunctivitis.
- Keratitis.
- Stye.
- Orbital cellulitis.
- Red eye.
- Blepharitis.

Vascular

- Floaters.

Neurological

- Acute glaucoma.
- Giant cell arteritis.

RARE PRESENTATIONS

Ruptured globe.

IMMEDIATE CHECK

- **Severe pain?**
- **Can the patient see?**
- **What is the state of the cornea?**

HISTORY

- Describe the mechanism of injury.
- If something struck the eye, what was it and at what velocity did it strike?
- Has any first aid been performed?
- What was the time of onset?
- Are one or both eyes affected?
- What was the prior visual function?
- Has any prior surgical procedure been performed on the eye?
- Contact lens wearer (have they been removed?).
- Past medical history (particularly diabetes).
- Family history.
- Current medications.
- Allergies.
- Social history.
- Tetanus status.

EXAMINATION

Look

Examination of the eye should be approached in a systematic and methodical way to consider each structure in turn.

Eyelashes

- Trichiasis (ingrowing eyelashes).

Lids and orbits

- Eyelid oedema.
- Redness.
- Discharge.
- Lids sticking together.
- Crusting.
- Ectropion: the eyelid margin is turned outwards, often with a sagging lower lid.
- Boil (furuncle of eyelash).

Pupils

- Size.
- Shape.
- Reaction to light.
- Relative afferent papillary defect.

Conjunctiva

- Conjunctival oedema.
- Injection.
- Bloodshot eye.

Cornea

The most vulnerable part of the outer eye and the most sensitive.

- Watering.
- Photophobia.
- Infiltrates – white spots.
- Ulcer on the cornea.
- Corneal thinning.

Anterior chamber

- Collection of blood (hyphaema).

Feel

- Irregularity of bony margin may be palpated.
- Digital palpation of the eyeball should only be performed by an experienced practitioner.

Movement

There are six extraocular muscles attached to each eye, giving a full range of movement. Each muscle is supplied by one of three cranial nerves: oculomotor III, abducens VI, trochlear IV.

Ask the patient to keep their head still while following a slowly moving target with their eyes (right, up and right, up, up and left, left, down and left, down, down and right) while looking for any restrictions in the normal range of movements of one or both eyes.

Note the pupil reaction when light is directed into each eye one at a time. A slow or absent reaction is not normal.

Swing the light from one eye to the other and note the reaction of each eye. Both pupils should do the same thing at the same time. The swinging flashlight test is done primarily to detect an afferent papillary defect. Any difference should be noted and could indicate a problem with the nerve connection between the eye and the brain.

INVESTIGATIONS

The ophthalmoscope, for examining the posterior segment of the eye including the optic nerve and peripheral retina, is often used to demonstrate a red reflex through the pupil, indicating clarity of the optic media.

A slit-lamp microscope provides a highly magnified three-dimensional view of the surface of the eye. Eye disease cannot be accurately diagnosed without a slit-lamp examination.

Visual acuity

This is absolutely essential, even if only a rough guide.

Usually performed using a Snellen chart with the patient standing six metres away. The patient covers one eye and reads aloud the letters on the chart, beginning at the top and moving towards the bottom. The smallest row of letters that the patient reads accurately determines visual acuity in the uncovered eye. The test is repeated on the other eye. Visual acuity can be expressed as 6/6.

For patients unable to read a Snellen chart, assess using the criteria shown in Table 30.1.

Table 30.1 Visual acuity

Name	*Abbreviation*	*Definition*
Counting fingers	CF	Able to count fingers held at ½ m distance
Hand motion	HM	Able to detect hand movement at ¼ m distance
Perceives light	PL	Able to perceive torch light when shone into eye
No light perception	NLP	Blindness

MANAGEMENT OF EYE INJURIES

Chemical injuries

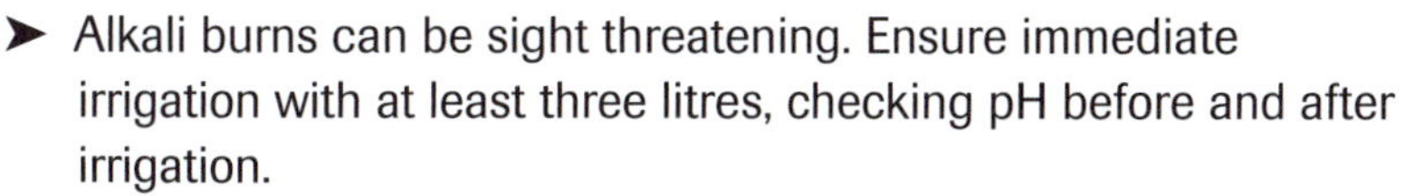

- Alkali burns can be sight threatening. Ensure immediate irrigation with at least three litres, checking pH before and after irrigation.
- Local anaesthetic eyedrops facilitate irrigation, preventing excessive blepharospasm.
- Check pH of eye.
- Severity is assessed by the degree of corneal opacity and limbal ischaemia (whiteness around the cornea).
- Refer urgently to an ophthalmologist.

Ruptured globe

Small penetrating injuries can be easily missed so careful examination is essential.

- Any penetration of the eyelids should raise suspicion of a globe injury.
- History of a projectile injury or a severe blunt trauma (consider flake of metal).
- On examination, reduced eye movements, subconjunctival haemorrhage and soft globe.
- Do not use force to examine the globe and stop further manipulation of the globe.
- Place a protective shield over the eye, not a pad.
- Keep patient nil by mouth for surgical repair.
- Analgesia and antiemetics are very important as vomiting will put further pressure on the injured eye.
- Consider the need for tetanus immunisation.
- Refer urgently to an ophthalmologist.

Corneal abrasions

- Instil local anaesthetic eyedrops in order to examine the eye.
- Fluorescein will stain an abrasion green and is particularly clear in a blue light.
- Avoid excessive use of local anaesthetic drops for painful corneal conditions as it may delay healing.

Subtarsal foreign body

- A piece of grit may have entered the eye and not be seen on ordinary inspection.
- Evert the eyelid.
- Remove grit with a finger or a cotton bud.
- Insert antibiotic ointment.

Corneal foreign body

- Extremely painful.
- Instil local anaesthetic drops (apply eye patch afterwards for protection).
- Steady eyelids of supine patient with one hand.
- Ask patient to fix their gaze on an object.
- Remove FB with a sterile hypodermic needle.
- Insert antibiotic ointment.
- However, if the eye is still sore, it will heal faster if padded for a day or two and seen in a review clinic or referred to an ophthalmologist.

Hyphaema

This is a collection of blood in the anterior chamber of the eye.

- Must rule out globe rupture or fractures.
- Examine the anterior chamber and do a retinal examination.
- Hyphaema is often associated with a corneal abrasion.
- Shield the affected eye.
- Refer to an ophthalmologist.

Black eye

- Open swollen eyelids digitally.
- Check the integrity of the cornea, depth of anterior chamber and whether or not it contains blood (hyphaema).
- Compare the pupil to the opposite side; does it react?
- Irregularity of the bony margin may be palpated.
- Always X-ray if 'blow-out' is suspected. Maxillofacial referral may be required.

Eyelid lacerations

- Take a careful history.
- Assume every lid laceration is associated with a globe laceration until proven otherwise.
- The most serious of these are those that involve the lid margin, particularly at the medial end of the lower lid where the lower lacrimal canaliculus may be involved.

- Careful repair is needed to avoid notching. Refer to ophthalmologists.
- Systemic antibiotics.
- Tetanus prophylaxis.

Open eye trauma

- Check visual acuity.
- Displacement of the iris or pupil should suggest the possibility of open eye trauma.
- Exclude the presence of an intraocular FB.
- Always X-ray to exclude an intraocular FB. The chance of blindness and losing the eye increases rapidly while the FB remains. The entry wound may be surprisingly difficult to see.
- Refer to an ophthalmologist.

Orbital trauma

- Blunt trauma to the orbit can result in swelling, bruising and fractures.
- Orbital haematomas can produce proptosis and corneal exposure and an increase in intraocular pressure.
- Suspect an orbital blow-out fracture if there are restricted eye movements with pain, double vision and eyelid swelling after blowing nose.
- X-ray.
- Ice pack for orbit for 24–48 hours.
- Broad-spectrum antibiotics.
- Ask patient not to blow the nose.
- Referral to ophthalmologist, maxillofacial team and neurological team if needed.

Retinal detachment

- Apart from myopia, trauma is the other cause of detachment.
- Patient will have experienced sudden deterioration of vision, floaters and flashing lights.
- Check visual acuity.
- Urgent referral to an ophthalmologist.
- Treatment is always surgical.

MANAGEMENT OF EYE INFECTIONS

Conjunctivitis

Bacterial conjunctivitis

- Almost always affects both eyes.
- The eyes are red, gritty and sticky with pus-like discharge.

- Lid eversion shows papillae (small, pink cobblestone-like lumps).
- No need to take microbiology swabs.
- Treat with topical antibiotic every two hours for five days.
- Warn the patient that the condition is contagious.

Viral conjunctivitis

- Often caused by the common cold virus.
- One or both eyes become red.
- Clear watery discharge with no pus.
- Lid eversion shows follicles which look like small, grey grains of rice.
- No treatment is of benefit; the infection will resolve with time.
- Warn the patient that the infection is highly contagious until the redness subsides.

Allergic conjunctivitis

- Most commonly occurs in patients with asthma, eczema or hay fever.
- Itching in one or both eyes.
- No discharge or a watery sticky discharge.
- Lid eversion may show papillae.
- Contact lens wearers should see their prescriber.
- Steroid eye drops may help but should only be prescribed on the advice of an ophthalmologist.

Red eye

- One of the most common eye symptoms.
- Important to recognise the severity of a red eye (distinguish between a good and bad red eye).
- Bad red eye is one red eye (rarely bilateral) of unknown cause with one or more of the 'five Ps':
  - pain
  - photophobia
  - poor vision
  - pus in the cornea or anterior chamber
  - pupil abnormality.
- Any patient with a red eye and one or more of the five Ps must be referred immediately and urgently to an ophthalmologist.
- Not every red eye is conjunctivitis.
- The underlying cause of bad red eye, glaucoma/iritis, can only be diagnosed using a slit-lamp and measurement of intraocular pressure.

- Good red eye is diagnosed when one or both eyes are red but there is no pain or photophobia and the eyes are otherwise normal. The underlying cause could be viral, allergic or bacterial conjunctivitis, dry eyes or blepharitis.
- However, refer if the red eye does not improve in two weeks or if it develops into a bad red eye at any stage.

Blepharitis

- A chronic, mild inflammation of the eyelids.
- The eyelid margins appear slightly reddened and thickened, with crusting or matting of the eyelashes.
- The eyes themselves may look normal or slightly red.
- The cause is a blockage of the eyelids' oil glands.
- Gentle cleaning of the lid margins twice daily with a cotton bud dipped in baby shampoo will help to alleviate symptoms.
- Patients may also have dry eyes, in which case prescribe lubricating eye drops.
- Refer to ophthalmologist if these measures do not help.

Orbital cellulitis

- Bacterial infection of the orbital soft tissue, which usually spreads to the orbits having started as infection in the paranasal sinus.
- Main complaint may be pain and double vision or blurred vision.
- Examination usually shows fever, red eye, mild to severe proptosis and limited eye movements.
- Sluggish pupil or relative afferent papillary defect (RAPD).
- Secondary meningitis or encephalitis can occur.
- May be life threatening and requires referral and admission.

Dacryocystitis

- Presents as a mass close to the lower lid.
- The patient develops a tense, red, painful swelling inferior to the medial end of the lower eyelid.
- It is due to infection of an obstructed lacrimal sac.
- Urgent ophthalmic referral is required.

Stye

- This is a small, pimple-like infection that may develop around the base of an eyelash (furuncle).
- Removal of the offending lash may cure the problem.
- If localised skin redness occurs, a short course of antibiotics may be given.

Keratitis

- Keratitis is an inflammation of the cornea.
- Presents as a painful red eye with reduced visual acuity.
- The conjunctiva is often inflamed.
- Discharge is often watery. Photophobia is common.
- Fluoroscein readily demonstrates any ulceration.
- Refer the same day to ophthalmology.
- Risk factors for developing keratitis include tear insufficiency, malnutrition, vitamin A deficiency, contact lens use, particularly swimming with lenses in place.

MANAGEMENT OF VASCULAR PROBLEMS

Floaters are normal imperfections in the vitreous jelly. However, new onset of flashes and/or floating spots in one eye usually indicates possible posterior vitreous detachment, vitreous haemorrhage or retinal tear which may result in retinal detachment. Urgent ophthalmic referral is indicated.

MANAGEMENT OF NEUROLOGICAL PROBLEMS

Acute glaucoma

- Acute glaucoma is a sudden rise in intraocular pressure. Symptoms include eye ache/pain. Can be mistaken for a migraine.
- Blurred vision, sometimes with haloes around lights.
- The cornea appears cloudy.
- Diagnosis can only be made by testing the eye's intraocular pressure.
- More common in long-sighted elderly patients.

Chronic glaucoma

- Common and risk increases with age.
- No eye redness/pain.
- Patient is usually asymptomatic.
- Slow painless loss of vision.
- Central vision loss signifies severe disease.
- Referral to ophthalmology.

Giant cell arteritis (temporal arteritis)

Age related, affecting only adults over the age of 50.

- A sight- and life-threatening condition.

- Urgent treatment can avert blindness.
- Symptoms include headache and scalp tenderness.
- Bloods for FBC and ESR.
- Urgent referral for high-dose steroids.

SECTION 5
Primary care

CHAPTER 31

Respiratory conditions

COMMON PRESENTATIONS

- Upper respiratory tract infection (URTI).
- Pneumonia.
- Spontaneous pneumothorax.
- Pleural rub.
- Rib fractures.

IMMEDIATE CHECK

- Severe shortness of breath (SOB) with inability to talk in sentences.
- Respiration >20 breaths per minute.
- Peak expiratory flow <50% of predicted or best.
- Haemoptysis requires investigation.
- Remember to ask about travel. Atypical pneumonias are infrequent and tuberculosis (TB) rare but both can still present.
- Beware of persistent cough, weight loss and voice change in a smoker. An X-ray is required to exclude malignancy.
- The signs of an inhaled FB may mimic a lower respiratory tract infection (LRTI).

HISTORY

- Symptom analysis using **OPQRSTU**:
  - **O**ther symptoms and others unwell; SOB, hoarseness or chest pain
  - **P**rovocation/palliation; what brings the cough on? What relieves it?
  - **Q**uality/quantity; patient's description, e.g. rattling, is it productive? Type of sputum: amount, colour, smell, consistency, blood

- Region, radiation and recurrence
- Severity: is it keeping you awake at night? Does it cause you pain? Use the pain scale if appropriate
- Time and temporal: when did it start? Is it worse at different times of the day or night?
- **U**: What do you think is wrong?

➤ Relevant past medical history, i.e. respiratory disease, e.g. asthma, TB, pneumonia and hospitalisations, particularly intensive therapy unit (ITU) admissions for asthma.

➤ Current health: medication, allergies.

➤ Psychosocial: smoking, illicit drugs, occupation and travel.

➤ Family history: TB, asthma, allergic disorder.

EXAMINATION

General approach

➤ Ensure comfort, dignity and privacy.

➤ Examination processes – inspect, palpate, percuss and auscultate (see below). Always compare with the other side.

Look

➤ Obvious signs of anaemia.

➤ Cyanosis.

➤ Inspect the pattern of breathing and look for lip pursing.

➤ Use of accessory muscles, nasal flaring.

➤ Position of trachea.

➤ Supraclavicular lymphadenopathy.

Listen

➤ Audible noises, i.e. wheezing.

Inspect hands

➤ Finger clubbing.

➤ Signs of smoking and anaemia.

➤ Peripheral cyanosis.

Inspect eyes

➤ Check for signs of chemosis (oedema of the conjunctivae which may indicate CO_2 retention).

➤ Anaemia, seen as pallor of the underside of the eyelid.

Check mouth

- Look at the sublingual area and the lips for the blue tinge indicating central cyanosis.

General examination of chest

Chest examination can be subdivided into four sections: inspection, palpation, percussion, auscultation.

Inspection

- Check shape and movement of chest.
- Observe any signs of chest or spinal deformity which may indicate chronic lung disease or congenital abnormalities.
- Identify masses, scars, rashes.

Palpation

- Check integrity of thorax.
- Identify any areas of tenderness.
- Further assess areas of observed abnormalities.
- Respiratory expansion and tactile fremitus.

Percussion

- Anterior and posterior examination.
- Always compare both sides.

Auscultation

- Listen for sounds generated by breathing.
- Listen for adventitious sounds, i.e. crackles, wheeze, pleural rub or stridor.
- If abnormalities are detected listen for the patient's spoken word or whisper.
- Listen for heart sounds and bruit.

INVESTIGATIONS

- Chest X-ray (CXR).
- Sputum.
- Baseline observations.
- Peak flow.
- Bloods – FBC.

MANAGEMENT

Always refer to local policies and guidelines. However, patients should be assessed using the British Thoracic Guidelines (www.brit-thoracic.org.uk/guidelines.aspx).

Pneumonia

Pneumonia is an infection which causes the alveoli and smaller bronchial tubes to become inflamed and fill with fluid. Both young and old get pneumonia – even the young and healthy. However, it is more common (and usually more serious) in the very young and the very old. About eight in 1000 people get pneumonia every year (British Lung Foundation; www.lunguk.org). Although it is a very common illness, be careful with the use of the term 'pneumonia' as it can cause undue anxiety and needs careful explanation.

- Most patients can be treated at home but about 25% may need hospital admission.
- Community-acquired pneumonias are treated with antibiotics (follow local guidelines).
- Ensure analgesia and encourage an increased fluid intake.
- Smokers must be advised to stop smoking.
- Rest is an important part of making a full recovery.
- Advise patients that feelings of tiredness and lethargy may last for a few weeks.
- Refer to GP for follow-up.

Spontaneous pneumothorax

- Oxygen therapy if required.
- CXR to confirm severity of collapse.
- Three classifications of collapse:
  - small, <15%
  - moderate, lung collapse halfway to the heart border
  - complete.
- Conservative management is common when the collapse is small as long as the patient's breathing isn't compromised. It is essential to arrange follow-up in the chest clinic within 7–10 days to repeat the chest film.
- Moderate and complete collapses should be referred to the ED team for aspiration and/or insertion of a chest drain in severe cases.

Pleural rub and rib fractures

- Isolated rib fracture requires oral pain relief.
- Multiple fractures or flail segment require referral to the ED team for further assessment including arterial blood gas, observation and oxygen therapy.
- Pleural rub requires simple pain relief and advice about deep breathing exercises. If there is a history of trauma, consider a chest X-ray to exclude rib fractures. Secondary symptoms may develop, including a productive cough, and the patient may require antibiotics.

CHAPTER 32

Sore throat

COMMON PRESENTATIONS

- Viral and bacterial tonsillitis.
- FB in throat.
- Peritonsillar abscess.
- Oral carcinoma.
- Laryngitis.
- Reflux.
- Common cold.
- Glandular fever.

IMMEDIATE CHECK

- Severe SOB with inability to talk in sentences.
- Drooling and inability to swallow own saliva.
- Change in voice.
- Stridor/difficulty in breathing.
- Significant history of a fever which is not resolving.
- Persistent symptoms which are gradually getting worse or intermittent in nature. Could lead to a suspicion of carcinoma of the throat.
- Inability to lift tongue or swelling to the sublingual area; consider Ludwig's angina (rare but can occur).
- Sudden onset of change in voice and inability to swallow could indicate epiglottitis. This is rare in adults.
- Obstruction due to peritonsillar abscess (quinsy).

HISTORY

- Symptom analysis using **OPQRSTU:**
  - **O**ther symptoms and others unwell; SOB, change in voice
  - **P**rovocation/palliation; what makes it worse? What relieves it?
  - **Q**uality/quantity; patient's description, e.g. any discharge from throat including colour and consistency, any blood noted, smell from breath
  - **R**egion, radiation and recurrence
  - **S**everity: is it keeping you awake at night? Use the pain scale if appropriate
  - **T**ime and temporal: when did it start? Is it worse at different times of the day or night?
  - **U**: What do you think is wrong?
- Relevant past medical history, i.e. recurrent tonsillitis or history of admission for incision and drainage (I&D) of abscess.
- Current health: medication, allergies.
- Psychosocial: smoking, alcohol use, dental history, occupation and travel.
- Family history: allergic disorder.
- Pets at home.
- Seasonal symptoms.

GENERAL APPROACH

- Ensure the patient is comfortable.
- Observe for any obvious swelling, abnormalities, inability to swallow.
- Change in voice.
- Acute SOB.
- Obvious pain.
- Halitosis.
- Dehydration.

EXAMINATION

Ask patient to remove dentures, if fitted, and examine mouth systematically (use a bright torch): tongue, hard and soft palate, tonsillar fossa, gingivolabial/gingivobuccal sulci, floor of mouth, undersurface of tongue, as follows.

Inspection

- Check the hard and soft palates.
- Identify the uvula and ensure it is not deviated or swollen.
- Visualise the tonsils and check for exudate, ulceration and signs of abscess formation.

- Assess whether tongue is swollen or painful and that person has normal movement.
- Ensure no FB is visible to the eye.

Palpation

- Feel for tenderness or enlargement of the lymph nodes.
- Check for signs of fever, i.e. patient warm to touch or obvious tachycardia.

INVESTIGATIONS

- Baseline observations.
- Throat swab if exudate seen, to isolate the causative pathogen.
- If suspicious of glandular fever, take blood for Paul Bunnell test.

MANAGEMENT

Viral and bacterial tonsillitis

Many patients attend in the belief that they need antibiotics for a sore throat. It is important to explain the likely causative factors and the difference between a viral and bacterial infection.

Antibiotics do not contribute significantly to a patient's recovery even when tonsillitis is caused by a bacterium (NICE 2008).

Over-the-counter treatment to control pain is recommended, including simple pain relief, throat lozenges and an increase in oral fluids. Always advise the patient to return immediately if breathing becomes difficult or they are unable to swallow fluids.

- Bacterial tonsillitis: always refer to local policies.
- Viral tonsillitis: analgesia and supportive measures.

Foreign body in throat

- Check for angio-oedema.
- Soft tissue neck X-ray if the bone or object is radio-opaque.
- If visible to the naked eye, remove with forceps.
- Refer to ENT if concerned.

Peritonsillar abscess

- Immediate referral to ENT for admission and I&D.
- Patient may require IV antibiotics, depending on local policy.

Oral carcinoma

Cancer of the tonsil is rare but often the first symptom is pain. Discuss with and refer to ENT specialist if concerned and unsure.

Laryngitis, common cold and glandular fever

- Increase oral fluids.
- Simple over-the-counter analgesia.
- Rest.

Reflux

- Over-the-counter antacids.
- Dietary advice: avoid trigger foods including alcohol, coffee, chocolate, tomatoes or anything with high levels of fat or spice.
- Smokers should be advised to stop.
- Overweight patients should be advised that weight loss may relieve symptoms.

Reference

National Institute for Health and Clinical Excellence. *Respiratory Tract Infections – Antibiotic Prescribing. Prescribing of antibiotics for self-limiting respiratory tract infections in adults and children in primary care*. London: NICE; 2008.

CHAPTER 33

Nasal problems

COMMON PRESENTATIONS

- Epistaxis.
- Nasal polyps.
- Rhinitis.
- Facial pain caused by sinusitis.
- Rhinorrhoea (runny nose).
- Sneezing .
- Loss of smell (anosmia).
- FB in nose (usually children).

> IMMEDIATE CHECK
>
> - Signs of airway obstruction.
> - Excessive nasal bleeding.
> - History of trauma with a deviated septum.
> - Unilateral polyps can be indicative of a carcinoma.
> - Alcohol-dependent, haematology and anticoagulated patients are at high risk of nasal bleeding.

HISTORY

- Symptom analysis using **OPQRSTU**:
  - **O**ther symptoms and others unwell; SOB, change in voice
  - **P**rovocation/palliation; what makes it worse? What relieves it?
  - **Q**uality/quantity; patient's description, e.g. any discharge from throat including colour and consistency, any blood noted, smell from breath
  - **R**egion, radiation and recurrence
  - **S**everity: is it keeping you awake at night? Use the pain scale if appropriate

  - Time and temporal: when did it start? Is it worse at different times of the day or night?
  - **U**: What do you think is wrong?
- Specific questions need to be asked in relation to the nasal problems:
  - any history of direct trauma to the nose, i.e. assault or even picking
  - history of previous surgery
  - seasonal or daily variation in symptoms
  - allergies/atopic disease.
- Relevant past medical history, i.e. recurrent nasal problems.
- Current health: medication, allergies, particularly anticoagulants and seasonal allergies.
- Psychosocial: occupation, alcohol and smoking.

EXAMINATION

Full nose examination assesses function, airway resistance and occasionally sense of smell. It includes looking into the mouth and pharynx.

Inspection

First look at the external nose. Ask the patient to remove glasses, if worn. Look at the nose from the front and side for any signs of the following.

- Size and shape.
- Obvious bend or deformity: a deviated nose is often best looked at from above.
- Swelling.
- Scars or abnormal creases.
- Redness (evidence of skin disease).
- Discharge or crusting.
- Check patency of each nostril.
- Offensive smell.

Using the otoscope and Thudichum speculum, inspect the nasal cavities for:

- inflammation and swelling
- presence of polyps
- open wounds
- evidence of bleeding
- FB, usually accompanied by an offensive unilateral discharge
- deviation or swelling of the septum.

INVESTIGATIONS

- Baseline observations.
- Bloods to check clotting screen and FBC.

MANAGEMENT

Refer to local policies.

Epistaxis

Epistaxis is a potentially life-threatening event when posterior as opposed to anterior from Little's area. The elderly are particularly vulnerable.

- Initial approach – follow ABC.
- Patients who are actively bleeding need full assessment and resuscitation.
- Apply pressure to the nose and ask the patient to lean forward. Ensure this is performed for 10–15 minutes.
- If bleeding continues, refer to ENT for management. Usually the anterior nasal cavity is packed with a nasal tampon or sponge. If this does not arrest bleeding, more advanced techniques such as compressive balloons or posterior packing may be needed. The patient will then need admission for observation and removal.
- IV access and routine bloods, including group and save.

Nasal polyps

- A nasal polyp is a mass of gelatinous tissue which usually forms from allergy.
- Allergic nasal polyps can be treated by topical nasal steroids or by surgical removal.
- Often endoscopic sinus surgery is needed for their removal.

Rhinitis

- There are two types of rhinitis – intermittent and persistent.
- The most common cause of rhinitis is a cold. Hay fever is another common cause.
- Antihistamines and sometimes steroid nasal sprays may be helpful.

Sinusitis

Most patients with acute sinusitis are treated in the primary care setting. Sinusitis can cause significant facial pain and headache. In managing sinusitis, the main aim is to treat infection and alleviate the severity and duration of symptoms, and prevent complications. If the symptoms are not resolving after one or more courses of antibiotics, the patient may need referral to ENT. Many cases of sinusitis are, however, mild and self-limiting.

- Patients present due to sinus discomfort and difficulty breathing.
- NSAIDs and nasal decongestant sprays can be prescribed.
- Steam inhalation can also relieve symptoms.
- If symptoms are persistent, refer back to GP and advise referral to ENT for further management.

Nasal foreign bodies

Nasal foreign bodies are relatively common among paediatric patients and may also be seen in adult patients, particularly those with learning difficulties. Common items include toy pieces, beads, paper and food items such as peas, beans or nuts. The patient may have a unilateral foul-smelling discharge, sneezing, epistaxis or pain. Small button batteries are of concern, as they can cause chemical burns, ulceration and ultimately septal perforation.

Only attempt removal if the object is visible and the patient is co-operative. Otherwise, refer to ENT.

CHAPTER 34

Earache

COMMON PRESENTATIONS

- Otitis externa.
- Otitis media.
- Impacted wax.
- FB.
- Perforated tympanic membrane.
- Mastoiditis.
- Trauma and barotrauma.
- Labyrinthitis.
- Tinnitus.

LESS COMMON PRESENTATIONS

- Basal or squamous cell carcinoma.

IMMEDIATE CHECK

- Severe pain.
- Abnormal gait.
- Vertigo/dizziness.
- Bleeding from the ear.
- Mastoid tenderness and inflammation. Consider mastoiditis if tender behind the ear, foul-smelling discharge or generally unwell.
- Elderly patients with unexplained earache – consider nasopharyngeal carcinoma.
- Sudden onset of sensorineural deafness.
- Progressive unilateral deafness with tinnitus could be an acoustic neuroma.
- Long-term exposure to the sun and lesions to the pinna which intermittently bleed should raise suspicion of basal or squamous cell carcinoma.
- Discharge from the ear with associated confusion or neurological signs.

HISTORY

- Symptom analysis using **OPQRSTU:**
  - **O**ther symptoms and others unwell; SOB, change in voice
  - **P**rovocation/palliation; what makes it worse? What relieves it?
  - **Q**uality/quantity; patient's description, e.g. any discharge from throat including colour and consistency, any blood noted, smell from breath
  - **R**egion, radiation and recurrence
  - **S**everity: is it keeping you awake at night? Use the pain scale if appropriate
  - **T**ime and temporal: when did it start? Is it worse at different times of the day or night?
  - **U**: What do you think is wrong?
- Specific questions need to be asked in relation to the ear problem:
  - any history of direct trauma to the ear, i.e. assault, use of cotton buds
  - unilateral or bilateral symptoms
  - any hearing loss; if so, the onset and rate of progression
  - any symptoms of tinnitus
  - otorrhoea
  - vertigo.
- Relevant past medical history, i.e. recurrent ear problems or history of previous ear surgery.
- Current health: medication, allergies.
- Psychosocial: occupation and exposure to noise at work. Any foreign travel or flights. Specifically ask about swimming.
- Family history: including deafness and use of hearing aids.

EXAMINATION

General approach

- Look at the patient as they enter the room.
- Observe for signs of pain and distress.
- Observe for signs of swelling and abnormalities including hearing loss, confusion, etc.
- Remember to compare with the unaffected ear.
- Observe for any signs of imbalance or vertigo.

Inspection

- Inspect the pinna, tragus, entrance to ear canal for lesions, scarring, shape, size and position.
- Observe for any external discharge, including smell.
- Observe any inflammation or swelling to the mastoid process.

Palpation

- Palpate the pinna and tragus for pain, warmth, oedema or altered sensation.
- Feel the mastoid process.
- Palpate the pre- and post-auricular lymph nodes for enlargement, pain and irregularity.

Use of otoscope

- Always check the unaffected ear first to identify the patient's norm and ensure there is no cross-infection.
- Observe the patient for pain when the otoscope is inserted.
- Inspect the ear canal, identifying any abnormal findings including wax, furuncles, pustules, discharge or FB.
- Identify the tympanic membrane; ensure it is intact and the cone of light is present.
- Identify the key structures of the middle ear, including the handle of the malleus, pars tensa and pars flaccida.
- Ensure no fluid level is seen behind the tympanic membrane.

INVESTIGATIONS

- Tuning fork tests including Rinne and Webber.
- Baseline observations to exclude sepsis.

MANAGEMENT

Observe local policies.

Otitis externa

- Treat with topical antibiotics with or without steroids. Ensure the patient is able to administer the drops and lies down on the unaffected side for 10 minutes to ensure the drops infiltrate the canal.
- Regular over-the-counter analgesia.
- Avoid contact with water, stop swimming and immersing head in bath or shower.
- In severe cases the canal will narrow and close. With this presentation, immediate referral to ENT is required for aural toilet to remove the debris and insertion of a wick.

Otitis media

- Oral antibiotics (refer to local guidelines).
- Regular analgesia.
- GP follow-up.

Impacted wax

- Wax-softening drops for 7 days.
- Avoid using cotton buds.
- Analgesia if required.
- GP follow-up after 7 days to determine if the wax has resolved.

Foreign body

- Many FB are removed under direct vision with a hook.
- Drown live insects in olive oil before removing.
- If any discomfort, distress or difficulty removing FB, refer to ENT to consider removal under general anaesthetic.
- Once the FB has successfully been removed, re-examine and ensure no structures in the external ear have been damaged.

Perforated tympanic membrane

- Most patients with a traumatic tympanic membrane perforation do not require any specific treatment as they usually heal spontaneously.
- GP follow-up to ensure the perforation has healed in four weeks; if not, referral to ENT for assessment and possible surgical repair.
- Strict dry ear precautions are recommended to prevent water from getting into the ear. Instructions to the patient include no swimming and the use of a Vaseline-soaked cotton ball in the affected ear during bathing.
- A hearing test should be performed after 2–3 months to verify that hearing has returned to normal.

Basal or squamous cell carcinoma

If suspicious of the diagnosis, urgent referral to ENT is required.

Mastoiditis

- Need to assess the risk of intracranial spread of infection.
- Refer immediately to ENT if suspicious.
- Patient will need admission for IV antibiotics.

Barotrauma and trauma

- PRN NSAIDs.
- Arrange ENT follow-up.

Labyrinthitis

- Antiemetics may be prescribed.
- If the patient is persistently vomiting and unable to move independently, referral is necessary.

Tinnitus

- Tinnitus is strongly linked to stress.
- People are prescribed sedatives, tranquillisers or antidepressants to help lessen the effect of the tinnitus.
- Normally these are more effective if prescribed together with ongoing counselling.
- Patients should be referred back to their GP for ongoing long-term treatment.

CHAPTER 35

Urinary symptoms

COMMON PRESENTATIONS

- Cystitis (lower urinary tract infection (UTI)).
- Sexually acquired infections.
- Pyelonephritis (upper UTI).

IMMEDIATE CHECK

- Rule out urinary sepsis.
- Severe pain.
- Pyrexia.
- Pregnant women.
- Elderly patients with clinical signs of infection.
- Recurrent cystitis.
- Treatment failure – antibiotics resistance is more common.
- Individuals who are immunocompromised or have diabetes with features of a UTI.
- People who have a long-term catheter and features of a UTI.
- People with an abnormal genitourinary tract and features of a UTI.

HISTORY

- Symptom analysis using **OPQRSTU**:
  - **O**ther symptoms and others unwell; SOB, change in voice
  - **P**rovocation/palliation; what makes it worse? What relieves it?
  - **Q**uality/quantity; patient's description, e.g. any discharge from throat including colour and consistency, any blood noted, smell from breath
  - **R**egion, radiation and recurrence

- Severity: is it keeping you awake at night? Use the pain scale if appropriate
- Time and temporal: when did it start? Is it worse at different times of the day or night?
- **U**: What do you think is wrong?

- Specific questions need to be asked in relation to the urinary problems:
  - dysuria, frequency and urgency passing urine
  - haematuria
  - length of symptoms
  - nausea/vomiting
  - temperature
  - discharge, sexual history
  - occurrence and treatment
  - age and pregnancy
  - previous renal history.

EXAMINATION

- Ensure the patient is undressed and lying down.
- Ensure privacy.
- Observe the patient for pain, discomfort and signs of tachypnoea.
- Examine the patient's hands for signs of koilonychia, leuconychia, clubbing or palmar erythema, all of which may indicate physiological disease.
- Initially check the conjunctivae for pallor which could be a sign of anaemia.
- Also check the sclera for jaundice.

Inspection

Observe the abdomen for any obvious abnormalities such as scars, masses and pulsations or abdominal distension.

Palpation

- Palpation of the abdomen should be performed in a systematic way using the nine named segments of the abdomen.
- Palpate the non-tender area first and observe the patient's facial expression for signs of discomfort.
- Perform superficial palpation to ensure the abdomen is soft and non-tender, and to rule out obvious masses.
- Deep palpation for the spleen and liver
- Palpate the kidneys for tenderness in the renal region.

Percussion and auscultation

- Check for organomegaly.
- Listen for bowel sounds and bruit.

INVESTIGATIONS

- Baseline observations.
- Reagent urinalysis.
- Human chorionic gonadotrophin in women (with patient consent).
- Urine microscopy.

MANAGEMENT

Always check local policies and procedures.

Cystitis or lower urinary tract infection

- Can be managed with a course of antibiotics and discharged home. However, the specific type of antibiotic prescribed will depend on local guidelines and recurrence of infection.
- Offer paracetamol or NSAID to relieve pain and fever.
- Urine alkalinising agents may relieve the burning sensation and discomfort but there is no clinical evidence of their therapeutic effect.
- Increase fluid intake and reduce irritants, including caffeine.

Pyelonephritis or upper urinary tract infection

- Follow local guidelines.
- Referral to specialty.
- Admission for IV fluids, antibiotics and analgesia.
- Ultrasound scan.

Sexually acquired infection

- If suspicious of a sexually acquired infection, advise the patient to self-present or refer directly to genitourinary medicine (GUM).
- GUM will fully investigate and provide support for the patient during treatment.
- If unsure, seek advice from ED clinician or on-call specialty.

CHAPTER 36

Emergency contraception

Post-coital contraception may now be bought over the counter but vulnerable patients, particularly underage girls, may still present to EDs and urgent care centres needing help.

HISTORY AND EXAMINATION

- Date of unprotected sexual intercourse.
- Other unprotected exposure since last menstrual period.
- Reason why she did not use contraception.
- Urine human chorionic gonadotrophin.

CAUTIONS

- Use with caution in patients with sickle cell disease.
- Risk of recurrence if previous deep vein thrombosis.
- If a repeat user, need one normal period before giving pill again.

CONTRAINDICATIONS

- Greater than 72 hours post exposure.
- Positive pregnancy test.
- Last cycle not normal.
- Missed/delayed period.
- Breast cancer.
- Unexplained bleeding.

CHILD UNDER 16 YEARS OF AGE

Every attempt should be made to persuade the young person to discuss her situation with a parent or older relative. If she refuses, assess her competency in terms of the Fraser guidelines. Act in the best interests of the child and if there is any suspicion of abuse, refer to the paediatric team immediately.

ADVICE FOR PATIENT

- Need to repeat dose if she vomits within two hours.
- To return promptly if lower abdominal pain occurs (?ectopic pregnancy).
- To use barrier method till next period.
- To attend GP/family planning clinic if period more than one week later than expected.
- Advise about residual effects: nausea, breast pain, headache.

DRUG INTERACTIONS

Drugs such as anticonvulsants, rifampicin, ampicillin, tetracyclines and griseofulvin may affect the efficacy of emergency contraception.

CHAPTER 37

Suspected deep venous thrombosis

> Painful swollen lower leg is a common presentation for which there may be a number of causes; it is, however, essential to exclude a deep venous thrombosis (DVT) as it is an important cause of morbidity and mortality. Long journeys (more than four hours) by plane or train are thought to cause a slightly increased risk of DVT, so consider this if there is a history of recent long-haul travel.

HISTORY

- Duration of pain and swelling.
- Site/side.
- Any chest pain or shortness of breath.
- Family history.
- Risk factors (see Wells Score below).
- Past medical history.
- Medications.
- Hormone replacement therapy/oral contraceptive.
- Allergy.

EXAMINATION

- Limping.
- Swelling, erythema, warmth and tenderness.
- Compare with asymptomatic limb.
- Measure both limbs, 10 cm below tibial tuberosity; significant swelling is defined as 3 cm difference between limbs.

INVESTIGATIONS

Wells Score

If D-dimer testing is available, use the Wells Clinical Prediction Rule to assess the probability of a DVT.

ONE point for each of the following.

- Entire leg is swollen.
- Active cancer (currently under treatment or treatment within six months).
- Paralysis, paresis or recent plaster immobilisation of the legs.
- Recently bedridden for more than three days, or major surgery within the last 12 weeks.
- Localised tenderness along the distribution of the deep venous system (such as the back of the calf).
- Calf swelling by more than 3 cm compared with the asymptomatic leg (measured 10 cm below the tibial tuberosity).
- Pitting oedema (greater than on the asymptomatic leg).
- Collateral superficial veins (non-varicose).
- Previously documented DVT.

Subtract TWO points if an alternative cause is more likely than a DVT. Clinical probability of a DVT with a score of :

≥3 high
1–2 moderate
<1 low.

For more information, visit www.patient.co.uk/doctor/Deep-Vein-Thrombosis-(DVT).htm.

Other investigations

- Pregnancy and the oral contraceptive pill also increase the risk of DVT and patients who are IV drug users are particularly at risk so maintain a high index of suspicion and if D-dimer testing is not available or practical, refer immediately for a medical assessment.
- Most departments have their own protocols/guidelines for the management of DVT which include duplex ultrasonography.
- If the D-dimer test is **positive,** follow local guidelines for management. Initial treatment is with heparin, unfractionated or low molecular weight, followed by oral anticoagulation. Outpatient treatment of deep vein thrombosis is safe and these patients are usually followed up by the anticoagulant clinic.

- If the D-dimer test is **negative** and other causes have been excluded, reassure the patient and advise them to return immediately or go to their nearest ED if they develop difficulty breathing, increased breathing rate or chest pain (these symptoms may suggest pulmonary emboli).

DIFFERENTIAL DIAGNOSES OF SWELLING TO LOWER LEG

- Superficial thrombophlebitis.
- Chronic venous insufficiency.
- Cellulitis.
- Ruptured Baker's cyst.
- Gastrocnemius muscle tear.
- Fracture.
- Haematoma.
- Acute arterial ischaemia.
- Lymphoedema.
- Hypoproteinaemia (nephrotic syndrome or cirrhosis of liver).
- Cramp due to statins. Whilst cramp will not cause swelling, it is often not appreciated that cramp can be caused by statins.

CHAPTER 38

Headache

Headaches are a fairly common presentation in emergency/urgent care settings but only a small proportion, 10–15%, are due to serious underlying pathology. Making a differential diagnosis between what is potentially serious and what is not can be difficult and for this reason, practitioners should request senior help early on if concerned. EPs need to be very familiar with headache 'red flags' (see below) to ensure they do not overlook important clues to serious pathology. A detailed history and examination is essential to an accurate diagnosis.

CAUTION

If as an EP you do not feel competent to undertake a full neurological examination then refer your patient immediately to someone who does.

PRIMARY HEADACHES

These are usually low-risk presentations corresponding to 80% of all patients.

- Tension.
- Migraine.
- Cluster.

SECONDARY HEADACHES

These are more serious and the following possible causes should be considered.

- Vascular subarachnoid haemorrhage, stroke, hypertension,temporal arteritis.
- Intracranial disorders such as tumour.
- Central nervous system infections, encephalitis, meningitis.
- Sinusitis, neuralgia, dental pain.
- Metabolic disorders.
- Poisoning – carbon monoxide, drugs overdose, substance misuse.

- Be aware of alcoholic patients and the elderly as they may have a chronic subdural haematoma.
- Any recent history of head injury or seizures.

SIGNIFICANT HEADACHE 'RED FLAGS'

- Sudden-onset severe pain, 'thunderclap', which reaches maximum intensity in seconds.
- Disturbs sleep.
- Early morning headache.
- Increased pain on coughing or sneezing.
- Severe pain that is different from previous headaches – 'worst ever'.
- Progressive pain over time.
- Pain in the occiput, or unilateral and always in the same area.
- Neck stiffness.
- Known immunocompromised status.

HISTORY

- New-onset headache, particularly occipital; consider intracranial bleed.
- In patients who have a past history of headaches, it is important to distinguish if this is different from the usual headache.
- History of fever, nausea, vomiting, photophobia, neck stiffness or seizure.
- Past medical history: headaches, migraine, neuralgia, glaucoma, hypertension, vasculitis.
- Medication history, any new medications.
- Allergy.
- Social history: if alcohol problems, consider chronic subdural haematoma and look for signs of recent trauma.

EXAMINATION

- Assess vital signs, including GCS; look for any evidence of head injury, scalp tenderness.
- Check visual acuity, pupil reactions, eye movements and papilloedema.
- Palpate sinuses for tenderness.
- Look in both ears for signs of infection.
- Examine skin for any rash.
- Do a full neurological examination, including cranial nerves (Chapter 9).

MANAGEMENT

- The management of the headache patient is dependent on the identification of life-threatening conditions. If there are no red flags, vital signs are within normal range and the patient settles with analgesia, discharge and refer back to GP for follow-up.
- If there are any red flags or you have any concerns whatsoever, request immediate senior review. Do not discharge the patient until reviewed by a senior ED doctor, middle grade or consultant.

Index